The One Thing That Changes Everything

A midlife reset for the woman who's ready to feel like herself again.

WRITTEN BY

Tina Haller

LiveLife**Happy** Publishing

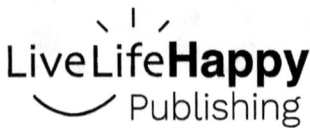

Published and Distributed in Canada by Live Life Happy Publishing.
www.livelifehappypublishing.com

Library of Congress Cataloging-in-Publication Data

Tina Haller

The One Thing That Changes Everything

Health, Fitness & Dieting > Women's Health > Midlife

Self-Help > Personal Transformation > Motivation & Self-Improvement > Eating Disorders & Body Image

Body, Mind & Spirit > Healing › Energy

ISBN: 978-1-998724-32-1 Paperback

ISBN: 978-1-998724-33-8 E-Book

Cover Design: Tina Haller

Live Life Happy Publishing

PUBLISHER'S NOTE & AUTHOR DISCLAIMER

This publication is designed to provide accurate and authoritative information concerning the subject matter covered. It is sold to understand that the publisher and author are not engaging in or rendering any psychological, medical or other professional services. If expert assistance or counselling is needed, seek the services of a competent medical professional. For immediate support call your local crisis line. The following book could contain actual events and experiences that the author has encountered in their life. However, some names and specific locations have been changed or omitted to protect the privacy and confidentiality of the individuals involved. The changes do not alter the story's integrity or its messages.

Table of Contents

PART ONE
Show Up Authentic with Integrity

PART TWO
Living By Your Core Values

PART THREE
Ask The Question That Changes Everything

Acknowledgements

No book is ever written alone.

While my name may be on the cover, every page carries the fingerprints of people and moments that shaped me, challenged me, and reminded me of what it means to live aligned.

And to the women I've had the privilege to coach and walk beside: thank you for trusting me with your stories, your struggles, and your hopes. You showed up fully for yourselves — putting your health first, staying curious, and opening to new perspectives.

Your courage and commitment are a living example of what's possible. You've reminded me again and again that transformation is never about perfection, but about permission — the brave choice to return to your true self.

To my family, who have loved me in both my driven seasons and my quiet ones: thank you for being my grounding place and my compass when the path wasn't clear. To my children, Matthew and Kaitlyn — the lessons, joys, and challenges of motherhood have shaped the woman I am today.

The insights within this book are rooted in those experiences with you, and who I am now carries the imprint of the journey we've shared. And to my husband — thank you for supporting me as I realigned to my truths, for holding steady even when it was hard, and for giving me the space to do the personal growth that now lives within these pages.

To those who read early drafts, offered thoughtful feedback, and helped me sharpen the message on these pages — thank you. Your honesty, insight, and care shaped this book in ways I could never have done alone. You helped me bring the heart of this work into clearer focus.

To my teachers, mentors, and colleagues who have challenged me to think bigger, dig deeper, and always return to integrity: I am grateful for the wisdom you've shared and the example you've lived.

And to you, the reader: thank you for showing up for yourself by walking through these pages. You are the reason this book exists, and my hope is that you feel less alone and more at home in who you are.

May these words ripple outward into your life, carrying ease, freedom, and the reminder that alignment is always within reach.

My Journey

By the time I reached midlife, I had already spent years chasing every solution outside of myself — the newest diet, the hardest workout, the supplement that promised a miracle — convinced I was just one formula away from finally feeling like myself again.

But no matter how much effort I poured in, my body kept telling a different story: exhaustion, restlessness, and a quiet knowing that the answer wasn't out there at all.

Then menopause arrived, and the shifts it brought didn't create my struggles — they magnified them. What I could once push through with willpower now left me depleted and questioning who I even was beneath the mask I had worn for decades.

That mask had been built from years of *shoulds* — who I thought I was supposed to be, how I thought I had to show up, what I believed I needed to prove. On the outside, it looked polished. On the inside, it left me restless and empty. The fatigue, the cravings, the fog — they weren't failures. They were whispers pointing to a deeper truth — *this mask isn't you*.

When I finally turned inward, I uncovered what had been

there all along — my authentic self. And here's what surprised me: authenticity carried its own frequency. It wasn't loud or flashy. It felt steady, grounded, and liberating — like the exhale after years of holding my breath. For the first time, my inner world matched my outer expression. The friction was gone.

That's when I realized health wasn't something to chase. It was the natural state that emerged when I stopped living for everyone else's expectations and began aligning with who I truly was.

Somewhere in that stillness, I saw the gap I had been living inside—the space between managing my life and actually inhabiting it. My body had sensed it long before I did. That awareness became my turning point, the moment alignment stopped being an idea and started becoming a lived experience.

The shift I had been searching for wasn't another plan or program; it was a journey back to myself. That realization changed everything. Once I stopped fighting my body and started listening, I saw how deeply my well-being was intertwined with my *Aligned Identity* — the place where who I am and how I live finally moved together.

Choices that once felt impossible became natural and my body seemed to respond differently, as if it could finally work with me rather than against me.

This book was born from that journey. It isn't another checklist or quick fix. It's my story of losing myself, finding my way back, and discovering what it really means to live aligned. My hope is that in these pages you'll find echoes of your own story, and permission to stop searching outside yourself — to rediscover the identity that allows you to move forward with clarity, energy, and strength.

What changed my life wasn't more discipline—it was alignment. That's the space where energy multiplies, health returns, and freedom begins. In the pages ahead, I'll show you how to create that same inner environment so your body can do what it's designed to do: heal.

So stay with me. This may not be your typical self-help book promising more energy or balance. It's something deeper — a new way to understand vitality itself. The kind that begins within, where alignment replaces effort, and your body finally feels like home again.

Introduction

Our bodies are complicated — layers of systems, signals, and stories, no two alike. And yet within all that complexity lies something beautifully simple: the body's innate ability to heal when provided with the right environment.

For too long, we've been taught that healing lives some-where outside of us — in the next prescription, supplement, or quick-fix promise. We've been told to chase balance as if it were something to earn or achieve. However, the truth is that beneath all the noise, your body has never forgotten the way home. It carries an ancient intelligence, a quiet map back to wholeness.

All it asks is space. Gentler rhythms. Deeper breaths. Conditions where safety can settle in again. When you create that space, balance doesn't have to be forced. It remembers. It returns.

You already hold more influence over your health than you realize. Every small choice — the food you eat, the way you breathe through stress, the moments you choose rest instead of pushing through — is a signal. Each signal either pulls you further from balance or brings you closer to it.

The Midlife Mirror

This becomes especially clear in midlife. The changes in your body often arrive alongside changes in every corner of life — children leaving home, aging parents needing more care, careers evolving or losing meaning, relationships shifting shape.

It can feel like the ground beneath you is moving in every direction at once. The hormonal transitions of this season may amplify the strain, but they're rarely the whole story. It's the *stacking* of it all — the responsibility, the letting go, the quiet question beneath it: *What now? Who am I in this next chapter?*

You keep holding everything together, but deep down there's a whisper: When is it my turn? When do I get to come first?

If that sounds familiar, let me assure you: you are not weak, broken, or failing. What you're experiencing is your biology speaking in its own language. Fatigue, restlessness, fog, or emotional swings are not random — they're your body speaking in symptoms. The more you push against them, the louder they become.

What if, instead of seeing these symptoms as problems to fix, you saw them as messages — your body's way of guiding you toward balance? Every signal has meaning. When you learn how to listen, the fatigue becomes feedback, the fog becomes information, and the restlessness becomes a call for alignment.

That's where your healing begins — not in doing more, but in understanding what your body is asking for.

The liberating truth is this: finding balance doesn't require dozens of new habits or another exhausting overhaul. It requires one choice — to align with the identity that's been within you all along.

It's like the principle from *The ONE Thing* by Gary W. Keller and Jay Papasan: when you focus on the one action that makes everything else easier or unnecessary, your life transforms. But instead of productivity, this one thing unlocks vitality itself — when who you are and how you live move as one.

In this book, that one thing is aligning with your true identity — moment by moment, choice by choice. When you live from that place — the version of you that is authentic, aligned, and whole — everything shifts. Your food choices feel natural. Boundaries hold without guilt. Energy steadies without endless hacks.

But none of this happens without commitment. Commitment is the moment you decide your well-being is no longer optional. It's choosing to stop outsourcing your power and start owning it. Commitment isn't just an idea — it's a quiet decision that changes your direction. And with that decision comes responsibility.

Commitment sets the boundary; responsibility is the first seed you plant on the other side. Responsibility doesn't mean blaming yourself for the past — it means owning the choices you make today. That's freedom: no longer waiting for someone else to decide for you but reclaiming your quiet authority to act.

From there, the real shift begins. Every decision — how you eat, move, rest, and respond — gently guides you toward alignment, or reminds you where you've drifted. It's not about perfection; it's about direction. And each aligned choice builds trust with your body, an energy shift that changes everything.

Sometimes that looks like:
- Reaching for nourishing food not because you "should," but because it supports the woman you've chosen to be.
- Saying no to one more draining obligation, even when your old self would have powered through.
- Going to bed when your body whispers for rest, instead of scrolling through another hour of noise.
- Pausing in a stressful moment to ask: *"What would my aligned identity choose right now?"* — and then honouring the answer.

Think of it like planting a single seed. You don't need to manage the whole garden at once. You plant one seed, water it, give it sunlight — and over time, that seed transforms the entire landscape.

In these pages, you'll discover:
- It can be surprisingly simple to create the right environment for healing through small, consistent shifts.
- The three ingredients that form the foundation of your aligned identity — your compass back to clarity and energy.
- Why your symptoms are not the enemy but signals — and how decoding them allows your body to guide you toward what it truly needs.

This book is not here to add pressure or rules. It's here to clear the noise, reconnect you with your body's wisdom, and remind you of what your biology has always known: healing is natural when you stop fighting yourself and start creating the conditions to thrive.

So let this be your invitation. A map. A new operating system. Because when you align with your true identity — your one thing — everything else changes. Not just how you feel, but how you live.

Key Terms for the Journey

Before we go deeper, here are a few words you'll see throughout the book. Defining them now will help everything feel clearer as we go:

- **Mask** — The learned, protective identity we perform to feel safe or accepted. It often looks polished on the outside, but it hides the real self underneath.

- **Alignment** — When your inner truth, values, and actions all move in the same direction. It's the opposite of being divided between who you are and who you think you *should* be.

- **Core Values & Non-Negotiables** — Your deepest guiding principles. *Core values* are what matter most to you at the soul level; *non-negotiables* are how those values take shape in daily life — the lines you no longer cross or compromise. Together, they are your compass and your boundaries.

- **Authenticity & Integrity** — These two work hand in hand. Authenticity is being true — showing up as who you are without disguise. Integrity is acting truthfully — the bridge between what you believe and how you live.

Keep these in mind as you read. They'll return again and again, each time with more depth, serving as anchors to help you navigate back to yourself.

CHAPTER 1

The Lion and
the Mask

The Protective Roar

There was always a part of me that wanted to roar like a lion. Whenever I felt threatened, criticized, or dismissed, that roar stirred inside me. Sometimes it came out in words, but more often it was inside — loud, fierce, protective. It was my body's quiet plea: *Don't see how small I feel inside.*

That roar wasn't only anger. It was survival. Beneath it lived the old beliefs I had gathered over the years: I'm not enough. I don't belong. My voice doesn't matter. The roar was my subconscious trying to protect me from the ache of those stories being exposed.

From the outside, it may have looked like strength. But on

the inside, it was fear — fear of being unseen, unworthy, or unsafe. The roar was my nervous system's way of saying: *I'm trying to keep you safe — even if it costs your peace.*

The Armor We Wear

When the roar no longer worked, I built armor. I kept moving, even when my body whispered to rest. I overperformed. I smiled when I wanted to cry. I said yes when every cell inside me longed to refuse. It lit a fire beneath me — the drive to prove, to perfect, to earn the worth I already had.

The subconscious is always scanning for danger, and when it senses threat, it builds protection. Mine took the shape of perfectionism, people-pleasing, and proving. From the outside, it looked like discipline and drive; on the inside, it was protection.

And here's the paradox: the lion and the armor were never enemies. They were guardians — created to keep me safe. But over time, they also kept me contained. They blurred my edges, muffled my voice, and drained my vitality. Because pretending, even for good reason, always costs more energy than being yourself.

Every polite smile, every silenced truth, every yes that folded over a quiet no became another stone in the pack I carried. Eventually, that pack grew heavy. It didn't just tire me — it pulled me away from myself, eroding confidence, dimming my spark. What once felt like protection had quietly become confinement — a cage made not of bars, but of old beliefs that forgot how to let me breathe.

Only later did I realize the roar was never rage—it was a boundary my body didn't yet know how to speak.

The Mask vs. the True Self

Here's the truth: the roar wasn't my real voice. It was a mask — a reflex, a shield built from fear rather than alignment.

Beneath it lived another self — the one buried under years of "shoulds" and quiet survival. She was grounded. Clear. Steady. She didn't need to roar to be heard or perform to be seen. Her presence alone spoke truth.

This is how the subconscious protects us: when life feels uncertain, it builds masks. Masks that whisper, *If I look strong enough, maybe I'll be safe. If I stay busy enough, perhaps no one will see my fear. If I keep pleasing others, maybe I'll finally be enough.*

But authenticity doesn't bargain. She doesn't need disguise. She knows her values and moves in quiet congruence with them. She doesn't wait for permission — she simply lives in rhythm with her truth.

It took me time to see this difference — to soften toward the lion that once protected me, to thank her for her loyalty, and then to let her rest. What remained was not noise, but stillness. Not defense, but clarity. A kind of strength that speaks softly — yet carries truth that never wavers.

When Midlife Magnifies the Mask

Here's the thing: midlife doesn't necessarily create these struggles — but it can turn up the light on what was already there. The signs may have been present for years, moving quietly beneath the surface: the tight smile, the swallowed truth, the long hours of proving when your body whispered for rest. For many of us, the mask softens the noise just enough to keep going.

But midlife, in its fierce honesty, can remove the dimmer switch. What was once tolerable may start to feel too loud to ignore. The mask that once felt light now presses down — dense, unyielding — and the effort to hold it in place may start to show in your body, your mood, your energy. What once worked — pushing harder, saying yes, holding it all together — can begin to fracture under the glare of change.

For me, the magnification came suddenly — through loss. My sister got sick, and within ten days, she was gone. No warning. No time to prepare. One moment we were talking about everyday things; the next, life stopped.

Grief has a way of stripping away illusion. In those days that followed, I watched time bend — everything that had felt important before suddenly felt small. Her death cracked open something in me that I hadn't allowed myself to see: all the ways I had been living on autopilot, pushing through, ignoring the quiet signals from my own body.

Her story was my mirror. She had always given so much — always showing up, always doing for others, always strong. And as I stood in the quiet after she was gone, I realized I was doing the same. I was surviving on endurance, mistaking resilience for worth, believing that if I could just keep it all together, I'd somehow be safe.

Losing her forced me to face what I had refused to acknowledge — that I had been living from my mask, not my truth. I was holding everything together but barely holding myself. And in that realization, grief became more than sorrow; it became a summons. A call to start honoring myself in the ways I had postponed for years.

It's not only your body that can shift, but the landscape of your life. Children leave home, and the house can grow both quieter and louder in its emptiness. Parents may age, and new responsibilities can appear — caretaker, decision-maker, the one who feels she must stay strong.

Careers can evolve or lose meaning. Friendships can drift or deepen. In the space between what was and what's next, an unsettling question often begins to rise: *Who am I now? What do I want this next chapter to be?*

These transitions rarely break you; they can simply reveal the parts that have long been waiting to be seen. Midlife can act like a magnifying glass, bringing overlooked truths into focus — the places where you may have overgiven, overperformed, or overridden your own needs. It's life's way of quietly whispering, *You can't keep living divided from yourself.*

And yes, biology can play a powerful role in this revelation. Hormonal rhythms can shift, the nervous system can recalibrate, and the body can become less forgiving of constant output. What once rolled off your shoulders can now linger longer. Cortisol can edge higher, blood sugar can waver, and sleep can grow lighter as your system stays alert instead of at ease. The exhaustion isn't weakness — it's wisdom. Your body is magnifying what your mind has ignored, quietly insisting on a new way forward.

Because every mask — the achiever, the peacemaker, the fixer — can require energy to maintain, energy that might otherwise be used for healing, repair, and renewal can instead be spent holding up an identity that no longer fits. The cost can be subtle but cumulative: less vitality, less clarity, less joy.

Midlife isn't punishment; it can be perspective. It can serve as a spotlight, revealing where your energy has been leaking and where your truth has been waiting to be discovered. The invitation remains the same: the old strategies — proving, pleasing, pushing — may no longer hold. As they begin to unravel, space can open.

And in that opening lives your greatest choice — to keep surviving behind the armor, or to step toward the self that's been waiting: steady, unmasked, and ready to lead the next chapter.

The Roar or the Truth

This can be the heart of the Lion and the Mask — a moment of choice. At first, it may come quietly. You might notice the tension: the impulse to keep roaring in defense, and the whisper that invites you to listen instead.

You may have quieted her, but your authentic self never truly disappears. She can remain as the quiet core of your *aligned self* — the part of you that knows what's true, even when you forget. She waits patiently beneath the noise, beneath the roles and expectations, beneath the polished answers. And when you stop performing long enough to listen, you may begin to feel her steady pulse — a truth that doesn't need to roar to be real.

And when you choose her — even in the smallest ways — the roar can begin to soften. The armor may start to loosen. The mask, at last, can grow thin enough to fall away. What remains isn't weakness. It's strength without struggle. A voice without fear. A life less ruled by survival and more guided by truth.

That's the shift — roar into truth, mask into authenticity, armor into freedom. And once you feel that freedom move through your body — even for a breath — you might start to recognize it everywhere. From that moment on, life doesn't need to go back to what it was; it begins to unfold in alignment with who you truly are.

CHAPTER 2

Beneath the Layers: Finding the Self We Left Behind

Midlife doesn't necessarily create these patterns — it can simply bring them to light. As estrogen and progesterone begin to shift, the body's stress system may have less buffer, so misalignment can cost more — and the signals might grow louder. To understand why this matters, we can look back to where these patterns often begin.

How We Learned to Hide

When we're little, most of us live as our true selves. We laugh when something's funny. We cry when we're sad. We move, play, and rest when our body tells us to. We are fully connected — instinctively whole within ourselves.

But as we grow, that natural rhythm can begin to change. We start learning the rules of the world around us — what earns approval, what draws disapproval. Somewhere along the way, we may begin to trade authenticity for a sense of belonging. Parents, teachers, and society show us what's "acceptable" and what's not.

Maybe you heard:
- "Be a good girl, don't be too loud."
- "Work harder, don't be lazy."
- "Put others first, don't be selfish."

Slowly, we start to adjust ourselves to fit these rules. We put on little masks to feel loved, accepted, and safe. At first, those masks help us navigate the world. But over time, they can accumulate — and with each one, a bit more of our true self becomes hidden.

We don't actually lose that self — it's still there — but it gets buried beneath years of "shoulds," roles, and expectations. Like a bright light covered by layers of fabric, it can feel dimmer, but it never stops shining.

Think of the subconscious as the quiet archive of your life — storing every lesson, every emotion, every moment you've ever lived. It hums beneath awareness, quietly influencing choices even when you believe you're steering the wheel.

As children, that archive is wide open — soft clay taking shape through every word and gesture we absorb. Brain science shows that during childhood, we spend much of our time in slower brainwave states — the same states linked to imagination, curiosity, and deep focus.

In that open state, we don't analyze — we absorb. If we hear "you're too much" or "you're not enough," the subconscious can store those messages as truth. If we watch our parents push through exhaustion, we might learn that rest is something to earn.

By adulthood, many of our behaviors — our reactions, habits, and decisions — are guided by those early imprints. It's why we might say yes when we mean no, overwork when we're tired, or reach for food or screens when what we really crave is rest. The conscious mind sets goals, but the subconscious still holds the map.

For a while, we can outpace that mismatch — running on discipline, caffeine, or sheer will. But eventually, midlife can hold up a mirror and quietly ask: *What still fits, and what no longer does?*

The hormonal changes, the sleepless nights, the feeling that something once steady has shifted — they don't necessarily break us. They can simply illuminate the cracks in our old survival patterns. And through those cracks, light begins to seep in.

Why It Can Feel Like We're Lost

When we live from old subconscious programs, life can start to feel heavy — like being on autopilot while carrying a weight we can't quite set down. We might find ourselves acting on reflex:

- Saying yes when we want to say no.

- Reaching for food, wine, or screens when our body is really asking for rest.
- Putting everyone else first and quietly leaving ourselves last.

On the surface, it might look like we're managing. But underneath, something deeper whispers: *This isn't me.*

That whisper can create a kind of tug-of-war between two selves:

- The **masked self**, guided by old programming, trying to stay safe through pleasing, proving, or pushing.
- The **aligned self**, the part that knows what feels true, steady, and right.

When those two pull in different directions, it can create fatigue, confusion, and restlessness — because living divided is exhausting.

And our bodies tend to register that divide. Each time we perform instead of express — saying yes when we mean no, smiling when we want to cry, proving ourselves when we're already depleted — our nervous system can receive the message: *It's not safe to be me.* That signal may quietly activate survival mode: stress hormones rise, the heart rate increases, the breath shortens.

This may sound familiar: you're mid-sentence in a meeting, confident in what you've prepared, when suddenly everything vanishes — the words, the flow, even your sense of control. Heat floods your chest, your hands tremble under the table, and you scramble to cover it up with a nervous laugh or a scribble in your notebook.

We'll revisit this story in Chapter 5, when we explore how alignment steadies the nervous system — and how she learned to speak without the mask.

That moment isn't failure. It isn't weakness. It's simply the body doing what it was trained to do: protect you. It's following old instructions that once ensured safety but now hold you back.

Sometimes those instructions show up as what we call *imposter syndrome*. On the surface, it feels like self-doubt or fear of being "found out." But beneath that, the subconscious may simply be replaying early beliefs: *I'm not enough. I have to earn my place. Don't let them see the real me.* Even when your conscious mind knows your value, your subconscious operates through survival patterns. To it, a boardroom can feel as threatening as a battlefield.

Your body is simply responding to the story it still holds. When that story whispers you're unsafe, your behaviors compensate — by over-preparing, over-explaining, or freezing in the moment. It's not weakness; it's protection. But protection has a cost — it drains energy that could otherwise be used for vitality and presence.

The good news? That same biology can be retrained. When your conscious mind starts aligning with new truths — *I am enough. I belong. I don't need to prove myself* — your body can learn it no longer needs to live in defense. The mask loosens. The nervous system steadies. Energy begins to return to what matters most.

This is the turning point: realizing the mask was never the

enemy — it was the protector. But protection isn't the same as freedom. The moment you begin to question those old stories, you create space for a new one — a story where your worth isn't conditional and your body doesn't have to stay on high alert.

The nervous system doesn't need perfection; it needs truth. Each time you choose alignment over disguise, you send your body a message it has longed to hear: *It's safe to be me.* That's the whisper of your authentic self returning — and the beginning of real ease.

A Shift in Perspective

Sometimes the hardest part of this journey isn't shedding the masks — it's how we interpret them. For years, many of us have viewed the fatigue, forgetfulness, mood swings, or restless nights as proof that something's wrong. But what if they're not flaws at all? What if they're signals — gentle nudges guiding you back to yourself?

When that perspective shifts, everything softens. Seeing your symptoms as feedback instead of failure allows compassion to replace judgment. The exhaustion wasn't laziness; it may have been your system begging for rest. The mood swings weren't weakness; they could have been whispers for deeper attention. The fog wasn't incompetence; it might have been your nervous system trying to protect you from overload.

This shift doesn't erase struggle; it simply meets it with tenderness. It opens the door to curiosity instead of criticism.

And through that doorway, you can begin to see what's been underneath all along — the self that has always been there, waiting to be heard.

Where Did Our True Identity Go?

The encouraging truth is this: we never actually lose our true selves. They don't disappear — they can simply become covered. Like a compass buried under layers of dust, the needle still points north, even if it's hard to see.

The child who laughed easily, cried freely, and trusted her body's wisdom is still within you. She hasn't vanished; she's been waiting.

The subconscious simply stored the old scripts: *Don't be too loud. Work harder. Don't be selfish.* Over time, those scripts can start to run on autopilot, shaping behaviors we never consciously chose. And yet — even when the mask feels firmly in place, your authentic self is still there, steady beneath it all, ready to re-emerge.

That's why glimpses of authenticity feel so freeing. A single aligned yes can feel like dropping a weight you didn't realize you were carrying. Your breath deepens. Your shoulders ease. Your jaw unclenches. Your whole nervous system exhales: *This feels right.*

These moments aren't coincidences — they're reminders. Proof that your body remembers what truth feels like. Invitations to return more often.

Your true identity hasn't been lost; it's alive and waiting — whispering through clarity, through instinct, through those fleeting moments of peace.

The Path Back to Alignment

At its core, this journey isn't about becoming someone new. It's about remembering who you already are. The self you thought was lost is simply waiting for space to breathe again. Beneath the noise and conditioning, you are still there — whole, steady, ready.

The return can feel unfamiliar at first. After years of people-pleasing, proving, or pushing through, the idea of living from your true self might sound uncertain. But the beauty is this: returning happens in small, steady choices. Each time you pause and listen for what feels aligned, you take one step closer home. Over time, those steps create a path you can trust.

Alignment isn't just emotional — it's biological. When you live from your true self, stress hormones can settle, sleep may deepen, and energy often steadies because you're no longer burning it through inner conflict. Your thoughts clear because you're no longer second-guessing every move.

Living in alignment can feel like shifting from walking against the wind to walking with it. Life will still have its weather, but instead of straining at every step, you begin to feel supported by the flow.

This is the work of this book — to help you uncover the

masks, quiet the old programs, and create space for your true self to breathe again. Because when you live from that place, everything can change — not just how you feel, but how your body responds, how your energy flows, and how your life unfolds.

When the mask begins to fall away, your body doesn't usually ask for more effort — it asks for ease. And from that ease, we turn to the next piece of the map — the ingredients that make alignment tangible.

CHAPTER 3

The Foundation of Alignment

The Three Ingredients

Coming home to yourself rarely happens by accident. It often unfolds in quiet moments — in the pauses between tasks, in the small decisions no one else notices. And while the path may look different for every woman, there are three core ingredients that can guide the way.

Think of them as the rhythm of alignment — the steady pattern that can help bring your life back into tune. When one of them drifts out of reach, life can start to feel off — like walking through fog or running on empty.

But when all three begin to work together, something inside can click into place. Your energy may ground. Your decisions might feel clearer. And your body can start to feel like an ally again — not something to battle, but something that walks beside you.

These ingredients aren't complicated. In truth, they're beautifully simple — yet returning to them can feel like remembering something you once knew by heart. Many of us have simply drifted from them, so rediscovering them feels less like learning and more like uncovering buried treasure.

These three ingredients form the quiet architecture of alignment. They can hold you when life feels unsteady and guide you back when you've lost your way. Imagine them as three roots of a single tree.

When all three are anchored, you can feel more stabilized, grounded, and alive. When one loosens, your balance may waver; the ground beneath you can feel less sure. But when all three take hold, something deep within steadies. Your breath slows. Your body feels supported from the inside out.

Each root nourishes a different part of you — authenticity feeds truth, integrity gives it form, and values keep it oriented toward what matters most.

Together, they create what I call the **Aligned Identity** — the place where your energy, integrity, and direction grow in the same soil, reaching upward in harmony. As you practice these roots, you may begin to feel your aligned self emerging — the lived expression of this identity in real time.

If authenticity is the breath and integrity the current, values are the compass. Together, they create your internal ecosystem. And at the heart of this ecosystem are three ingredients that make alignment possible.

1. Show Up Authentic with Integrity

This is where the peeling back can begin. Over the years, you may have tucked pieces of yourself away — to stay loved, accepted, or safe. Yet every mask asks for energy. Every act of pretending creates a quiet tension the body can hold in the shoulders, the jaw, the breath.

Authenticity invites the courage to let your true self be seen. Integrity steadies that truth — it's the bridge between what you feel inside and what you express in the world. One without the other can wobble: authenticity without integrity can scatter; integrity without authenticity can harden. Together, they can bring coherence — a felt sense of rightness.

When you live from that coherence, energy begins to circulate differently. Your nervous system can loosen its guard, stress hormones may ease, and vitality that once leaked into performance can flow toward repair. The body exhales. Life starts to feel more like something that fits — from the inside out.

2. Live by Your Core Values

If authenticity removes the masks, values can offer direction. Without them, it's easy to drift — pulled into obligations or roles that drain vitality and blur truth.

When you begin to name your non-negotiables — the values that truly matter, like protecting time with loved ones, honoring honesty, or safeguarding your health — the noise can quiet. You pause, feel for alignment, and ask whether the path ahead matches the life you actually want to live.

Values can become the calm beneath the waves. They anchor authenticity and give integrity a compass so that what you believe inside naturally starts to show up outside. Together, they form a living foundation of alignment — a space where energy can steady, stress can soften, and life can begin to move with you instead of against you.

3. Ask the Question That Changes Everything

Every decision — large or small — can soften when you pause and ask: *What would my aligned self choose?*

That aligned self isn't some distant version of you. She already lives within you, emerging each time your choices echo your truth. Not the exhausted self who runs on proving, nor the one who disappears into pleasing — but the woman whose decisions feel clean, light, and true.

Each time you ask this question, you step out of survival and into creation. One honest choice at a time, you begin to live from the steadier rhythm that's been waiting beneath the noise all along.

Why These Ingredients Matter

Together, these three ingredients can dissolve the exhausting tug-of-war that keeps so many of us spinning. They can reconnect you to the quiet core of who you are — until your true identity becomes the one leading the way.

Living authentically stops feeling like effort and begins to feel like ease — a steady rhythm your body can trust.

When these ingredients take root, they may:
   • Ease the tension your body has been carrying.

• Bring clarity to the moments that matter most.

• Build a grounded wholeness no mask could ever give.

The rest of this book will take each ingredient deeper — inviting you to explore authenticity, uncover your values, and use this powerful question in real time.

Because when these three roots begin to hold, the midlife shifts no longer define you. You stop fighting with yourself. You stop drifting. And you begin to live with energy, clarity, and freedom — not by force, but by design.

This is where the journey deepens — where rhythm becomes root, and alignment begins to live through you.

1

Part One

Show Up Authentic with Integrity

CHAPTER 4

The Mask We've Been Wearing

A Life Lived in Costume

There can be a strange kind of comfort in playing the part you've always played.

For years, I believed I was doing everything right — smiling at the right moments, saying yes when every cell in my body whispered no—pushing through exhaustion. Pretending I wasn't quietly unraveling inside.

From the outside, it might look seamless — career, family, health, all the boxes checked. But inside, it can feel like living in costume, cast in a role you never truly auditioned for.

Maybe you know that feeling. You wake, gather your "good-day" face, and step into the role of dependable mother, reliable colleague, patient partner — even when a quieter voice inside may whisper, *this isn't me.*

That's the mask at work. Not sequins and makeup, but layers stitched from years of *shoulds* and silent expectations. A smile that doesn't quite reach the eyes. A nod when the body wants to shake its head. A "yes, of course" that can turn bitter the moment it leaves your lips.

At first, the mask can feel light and easy. Like carrying a small purse. But season after season, more gets tucked inside: responsibility, guilt, the need to prove.

Then midlife approaches, and life can shift on multiple fronts at once — kids leaving home, roles at work changing or winding down, caring for aging parents, relationships evolving, a quiet *what now?* rising in the spaces once filled by schedules.

The strap that once felt sturdy may start to dig in. What once ran on willpower can begin asking more than the body or heart wants to give.

One day, you catch your reflection and feel a flicker of distance. The face is yours, yet not quite you. The eyes can hold a fatigue no concealer touches. The body that once bounced back now hesitates — slower, more tender. These aren't just symptoms; they may be signals. The body whispering what the spirit has long known: the mask isn't free. It's costing you.

And this is where the turning can begin — not with more effort, but with honesty. The quiet willingness to see the costume for what it was: not safety, not strength, but a covering that kept you from your own light.

As those layers loosen, the air may feel different — lighter, cleaner. The breath can move a little deeper. The weight you've carried for years may begin to shift — not all at once, but gently, as though life itself is exhaling with you.

This is the quiet relief of truth: realizing you don't have to perform to belong.

The Social Mask

We often learn early how to wear a mask. At school, it might have been the good girl — polite, agreeable, easy to manage. At home, the responsible one — smoothing tension, keeping the peace. Later, the roles can multiply: devoted partner, dependable employee, or an always-there friend.

Each role can earn approval. Each practiced smile may keep the waters calm. Slowly, the performance becomes familiar — almost comforting. We can forget where the role ends and the real self begins.

Here's the quiet cost we rarely name: masks teach us to turn down our own signals. The slight tightening in the chest when we agree to what we don't want. The knot in the stomach after laughing off a comment that landed hard. The restlessness that surfaces at midnight after a day spent swallowing words.

Each moment seems small, but together they can shape how the body learns to live — braced, alert, always managing. Over time, the mask doesn't just protect you from others; it can muffle you from yourself. It whispers that belonging is safer than truth, until you start doubting the sound of your own knowing.

Midlife often brings this pattern into focus. Hormones may shift, sleep patterns can change, and patience may wane. Add the real-life transitions — an emptier house, new financial realities, rethinking work or retirement, parents needing more, friendships changing shape — and the performance can feel heavier. What once helped you cope may begin to drain your system.

This isn't failure. It can be feedback — your whole system saying, *I can't carry this anymore.*

And that's where the turn may begin. Not by blaming the mask, but by seeing it clearly. It protected you when protection felt necessary. It helped you navigate when you didn't yet trust your own map. But now, life might be asking for something different. Less perfection, more presence. Less polish, more truth.

As the mask loosens, you may begin to hear yourself again — not the curated version, but the one underneath: steady, clear, quietly strong. That's the woman the world may have been waiting for.

———————— *The Identity Mask* ————————

Masks don't only cover our faces — over time, they can seep into our sense of self.

What begins as protection can slowly become who we think we are.

Initially, the mask is something we consciously put on. We smile when we're sad. We nod when we want to refuse. We say yes because no feels dangerous. With years of repetition, the seams blur. The performance can fuse to the skin. We may no longer know where pretending ends and self begins.

That's why so many women in midlife whisper, "I don't even know who I am anymore."

It's not amnesia. It's accumulation. Each role — daughter, partner, mother, professional, community-builder, caretaker — can layer over her voice until the sound of her own truth grows faint. She isn't gone — just tucked beneath years of *ought to* and *have to*, waiting to be uncovered.

Here's the tender paradox: the mask that once kept you safe can eventually hide you. People may see the perfected version — competent, composed, reliable — but miss the woman inside. In that invisibility, something can start to dim. First you stop feeling seen. Then known. Eventually, fully alive.

Midlife tends to pull this truth into the light. The old armor may crack, and what's been hidden can begin to surface. You catch your reflection and recognize the face but not the gaze.

In that moment, something inside often pauses — a breath, a beat, a quiet noticing.

The mask once offered protection, but now it may charge a price — connection, presence, vitality. Left untouched, the risk isn't failure — it's forgetting.

And here's the gift: what's forgotten can be remembered. The woman who laughed freely, moved instinctively, spoke without rehearsing — she can still be here. Beneath the performance. Beneath the polish. Beneath the years.

This isn't about ripping the mask off in one dramatic sweep. It's about loosening it, thread by thread, until the breath of the real self reaches the surface again — and the body recognizes home.

—— *The Quiet Cost of Holding It All Together* ——

There can be a quiet cost to holding it all together — not in terms of dollars, but in terms of energy.

Each time a polite 'yes' replaces the 'no' that was intended, a small current may leave the body. Each swallowed truth can tighten the chest and thin the breath. Each smile offered through the ache asks the body to pay quietly — like coins slipping from a purse no one realized had a hole.

Initially, you may not notice the cost. A little fatigue here. A restless night there. But the body keeps its own accounting. Every small self-abandonment can leave a trace: a knot beneath the ribs, a heaviness behind the eyes, a pulse that won't quite settle.

As midlife arrives, the price of pretending may grow higher. Hormones might not buffer stress the way they once did. Add the emotional load of life transitions — supporting a parent, navigating a child's launch, re-imagining career or purpose — and what sheer will once carried can be hard to sustain.

Your body isn't turning against you — it may be telling the truth. Fatigue isn't laziness. Brain fog isn't failure. Restless sleep isn't random. They can be signals — gentle red flags from within, whispering: *this life is costing too much.*

And here's the shift many of us discover: Just as pretense drains you, honesty can restore you.

Each time your 'yes' truly means 'yes,' your nervous system may exhale. Each time you speak a truth, even a small one, the body can receive it like oxygen. Every boundary kept is a deposit. Every moment your inner world matches your outer one, energy can flow back in instead of leaking out.

"It was like unclenching a fist I didn't know I'd been making," one woman said after her first unapologetic no.

That isn't magic — it's biology aligning with truth.

The shift is often immediate: the first honest no, the first breath that reaches the belly, the first moment you stop performing and start living. That's energy returning home.

Living this way may not erase the storms of midlife, but it can change how you move through them. You stop running on borrowed fuel. You stop paying the tax of pretending. You begin to feel a steadier kind of power — quiet, renewable.

Room for the Real You

There may come a moment when holding the mask in place feels like holding your breath. You can live that way for a while — performing, pushing, pretending — but not fully. Not freely.

Every forced smile, every polite yes, every truth swallowed for ease can tighten something inside. It's like moving through the day with a band around your chest — functioning, but never quite breathing.

Authenticity is what can loosen that band. It doesn't require grand gestures or dramatic reveals. It often begins with the smallest release — an exhale you didn't realize you were holding.

It shows up quietly: admitting, "I don't know." Resting instead of pushing. Letting laughter escape unfiltered and real. Each honest moment cracks a window in a stale room. The air shifts. The light changes. Life moves again.

Authenticity doesn't mean revealing everything. It can simply mean no longer betraying yourself — letting what you feel inside align with what you allow to be seen outside.

When those match, the body usually knows. Shoulders drop. Jaw softens. Breath deepens. It's less effort—more remembering.

You don't have to think your way into authenticity — you can breathe your way into it. Each time your words match your truth, the body takes a deeper inhale.

That's the invitation of this season: to breathe again, fully and freely. To stop gasping through performance and start inhaling your own presence. Authenticity isn't a skill to master. It can be oxygen. And the more you breathe it, the more alive you may feel.

When the Mask Starts to Loosen

Think about the last time someone asked, *"How are you?"* and before you even paused to check, the words *"I'm fine"* slipped out. Even when you weren't.

That quiet reflex — that's the mask smoothing things over.

At first, it feels harmless — a shortcut through the noise, a way to get through the day. But over time, the cost adds up.

If you pause for a moment, you can feel it. The weight of always holding it together. The way it tightens across your face, keeps your smile in place, and rests heavy across your chest.

Now imagine loosening it — just a little. Like unhooking

a strap that's been pressing against your skin all day. Feel the relief as it slips away.

The air feels cooler. Your shoulders sink. Your jaw softens. And for the first time in what feels like forever, your breath moves freely.

In that moment, you may catch a glimpse of the real you — not the role you've been performing, not the polished version you've practiced, but the steady, unmasked you, finally able to exhale.

Living from your deepest truth doesn't mean opening every chapter to the world. It simply means you stop betraying yourself. Your yes means yes, your no means no, and your body no longer has to carry the cost of performance.

This is the deeper invitation: living unmasked isn't about fearlessness — it's about gentleness with truth. It's creating a life where your body and your choices move together, not in opposition. Each time you practice it — one boundary, one honest answer, one deep breath — you can clear the path back to yourself. And over time, that path begins to feel like home.

Here's the beautiful part: when the weight of masks begins to lift, your choice often expands. Fear can quiet. Obligation may loosen its grip. Clarity rises — reshaping how you relate, how you move through your days, and how your energy is spent.

That kind of clarity can open gentle doors — to growth that feels natural, to relationships that nourish, to experiences that align with what matters most. Living unmasked isn't just relief; it's aliveness. It returns your energy to what feels true — to shaping a life that fits like your own skin.

And when authenticity joins hands with integrity, the energy that once drained into old roles can flow back to you. It gathers. It steadies. It begins to fuel a life that moves with you — not against you.

The Energy of Alignment

Here's the beauty: you can often feel the shift almost immediately.

The first time you say no and mean it — the body exhales. The first truth spoken steadies your breath. The first moment without the mask — energy returns.

It isn't magic. It's the body remembering what truth feels like — the soft sigh of recognition after years of holding its breath.

When life drifts out of alignment, it's rarely just one thing that feels off. It ripples through your whole system. The calendar fills, the house grows quiet, a parent's health falters, work loses its spark, the body changes its rhythm. The world begins to feel louder, and the old strategies that once helped you cope may start to feel thin.

But these changes aren't punishment — they're conversation. Your body and life are speaking in a new rhythm, inviting you to slow down enough to listen.

Pause. Rest a hand over your heart. Feel the quiet *yes* beneath your palm.

One small misalignment can set others off course — a choice here, a habit there — until the whole system hums out of tune. That's why what once felt like a minor stressor can now land heavier. Midlife doesn't create the dissonance; it simply amplifies what's been asking for your attention all along.

Alignment changes the rhythm. When your choices match your truth, the leaks begin to close. Stress hormones settle. Digestion softens into ease. Sleep deepens. Energy begins to circulate instead of scatter.

The body moves from survival into restoration — clarity, vitality, and flow.

Think of it like a house with frayed electrical wiring. Every time the current leaks, the lights dim and the system strains. Integrity is the rewiring — clearing the circuits so energy flows clean again. The house brightens, not from adding more, but from losing less.

And in that quiet moment, you recognize it — the shift that changes everything.

I've seen women feel this almost instantly. One said, "The moment I said no without a story behind it, my whole body exhaled—like my nervous system finally believed me." Another shared that after setting a much-needed boundary, she slept through the night for the first time in months.

It's no coincidence — that's what happens when alignment quietly turns the current back on.

And here' the more profound truth: authenticity and integrity create the inner environment your midlife body and life have been asking for — a calm ground where nourishment, movement, rest, and renewal can finally take root.

Alignment isn't an idea. It's your power grid. Once the current flows clean again, you can see how dim the lights once were — and how naturally everything begins to move with you.

Living Unmasked

Living unmasked doesn't require a grand reveal. It begins with the smallest daily choices — the pauses that either keep the mask firmly in place or allow it to slip away.

Micro-betrayals keep the mask snug — each polite yes given against your truth, each smile that hides frustration, each silence that swallows what needs to be spoken. Every small act leaves a trace in the body: shoulders tightening, sleep unsettled, muscles holding tension that never quite releases.

But one pause can interrupt the pattern. A single breath before you answer signals to the nervous system, *I'm safe now.* That breath opens a new possibility — a moment of choice.

Truth lifts the mask. Your body exhales when your words and reality finally align. Even a quiet confession — "I don't know," "I need rest," "That doesn't work for me" — tells your system it's safe to be seen. Shoulders drop. Breath deepens — energy steadies.

Safety is what makes unmasking possible. The mask loosens first where it feels safest — with a trusted friend, in a private journal, even alone before the mirror. Each time your body learns that honesty doesn't equal danger, that safety expands into more corners of your life.

Quiet wins lift the mask, piece by piece. The first no without guilt. The first unfiltered laugh. The first time 'I'm fine' becomes 'Actually, today feels heavy.' These aren't small moments. They're messages to your nervous system: *this is who I am.*

Living unmasked isn't about fearlessness; it's about honesty

— a quiet return to yourself. Each act of truth realigns your biology and your being. Over time, the mask doesn't just loosen; it falls away. What's left isn't weakness, but the calm power of freedom — the steady aliveness that comes from no longer living at odds with yourself.

Unmasking is only the beginning — a quiet turning toward truth. Now that you've glimpsed the weight you no longer need to carry, the path ahead invites you to breathe more freely, to live in the ease of what's real. That's where we go next: into the calm power of authenticity.

Notice how even reading these words might slow your breath — that's integrity already beginning to land in the body.

TRY THIS: ONE BREATH OF TRUTH

Tonight, when you have a quiet moment, close your eyes and take a single deep breath.

Let it move through you — unhurried, steady.

Then ask gently, Where did I wear the mask today? Maybe it was the easy "I'm fine" when you weren't. Perhaps it was the nod when every part of you wanted to say no. Maybe it was the silence that held back what needed to be said.

Take another breath. Ask, Where today did I let the mask slip, even for a moment? Perhaps it was a laugh that came from somewhere real. Perhaps it was a clear 'no' that needed no apology. Perhaps it was a quiet, "I don't know," that felt like honesty.

Simply observe what unfolds as you recall each one — the softening, the release, the remembering. You don't have to fix or change anything. Awareness itself is enough to begin the repair.

Before you sleep, whisper one small truth you'll carry into tomorrow. Keep it simple. Keep it kind. One breath of truth at a time, you are teaching your body the feeling of home.

CHAPTER 5

Authenticity as Power Source

At its core, authenticity can be an invitation to stop negotiating with yourself. It asks, *Am I true to myself right now?*—and then lets your actions echo that truth. It isn't about spilling your whole story or living without fear; it's about staying with what's real.

Where masks can suffocate, authenticity often feels like oxygen. The moment you drop even one layer of performance, your nervous system may register it instantly: tightness drains, breath finds rhythm, energy moves. That relief isn't only emotional — it can be biological.

This chapter is a reminder that your truth isn't a liability; it can be your fuel. Practiced in small, daily choices, authenticity can create a steady power source no mask, role, or expectation can take.

— *The Day I Stopped Negotiating With Myself* —

For a long time, I lived in a full-blown courtroom drama — inside my own head. Every decision sparked a debate.

I'd decide to go to bed early... then immediately cross-examine myself about answering *just one more* email. I'd promise myself a peaceful walk... and end up deep-cleaning the fridge instead, because apparently, wilted lettuce is more urgent than my sanity.

It was exhausting — like being the lawyer, the witness, and the judge in a trial that never ends. And spoiler: there was never a verdict. Just recess... until the next round.

Back in Chapter 2, I shared the moment this chaos finally snapped into focus. It was a Sunday morning. After yet another night of overthinking and under-sleeping, I caught my reflection in the mirror — eyes puffy, soul tired — and whispered the most well-worn sentence in my vocabulary: **"I'll start tomorrow."**

But in that moment, something shifted. I realized... **Tomorrow was never coming.**

See, for years, *Monday* had become my imaginary rescue boat — always just out of reach.

"Next Monday I'll eat better."

"Next Monday I'll sleep more."

"Next Monday I'll finally take care of myself."

But every time I looked up, Monday was already waving goodbye, sailing off into the distance with my good intentions onboard. All that was left? More emails, more to-dos, and more reasons to postpone myself.

That Sunday, looking at my tired face, the truth landed simply: there is no boat. If I kept waiting for Monday, I'd still be waiting at 87 with a green juice in one hand and a to-do list in the other.

So... I stopped negotiating.

I realized authenticity wasn't a award I had to earn after enough pleasing, proving, or pushing through. It had to start now — in the tiny, ordinary choices that seem too small to matter but actually shape everything.

And here's the quiet surprise: Every time I stopped arguing with myself and just told the truth — I felt *better*.

My nervous system let out a sigh like, *"Finally, she gets it."*

My cravings got quieter.

My sleep got deeper.

And little by little, my body started to trust me again — not because I forced it into submission, but because I finally started showing up like someone who meant it.

That day, authenticity stopped being just a Pinterest quote or a self-help buzzword. It became a lifeline. From that point on, every honest "no," every boundary that didn't come with three paragraphs of apology, every moment I told the truth — was a step back home to myself.

And that's the invitation for you, too. Authenticity doesn't wait for perfect conditions, fewer emails, or the following Monday morning. It begins now. In the smallest, most human, most *you* choices.

Even if you still end up deep-cleaning the fridge instead of walking. (It happens.)

What changed wasn't my willpower—it was my willingness to tell the smallest truth and let it guide the next step.

The Heart of Authenticity

Authenticity isn't about oversharing or being "brutally honest." It's simpler — and far more powerful.

It's the moment you stop betraying yourself for approval. It's when your inner world and outer world finally match.

Your yes means yes.

Your no means no.

Your body stops bracing against performance and begins to breathe.

Why this matters in midlife: the whole ecosystem of your life can shift — roles at home, kids leaving for university, aging parents, evolving work or retirement, changing friendships, and yes, hormonal rhythms. With less buffer for chronic stress, small mismatches you once glossed over ("I'm fine," "It's nothing," "I'll handle it later") can echo louder through your system.

The body often keeps score. Cortisol, your stress hormone, can rise. The heart may quicken. Muscles can brace as if preparing for danger. Over time, even subtle self-betrayals may manifest as lighter sleep, foggier thinking, slower digestion, or a thinner patience. It's your body's way of signaling: *This mismatch isn't working anymore.*

Science echoes what your body already knows. Studies on midlife women show that as hormonal rhythms shift, the body can become more sensitive to stress and inflammation. Translation? Every false yes or swallowed truth weighs heavier than it once did — and every act of authenticity, no matter how small, carries an amplified benefit. One boundary honored, one truth spoken, one deep breath aligned with what's real can begin to steady the whole system.

That's why authenticity isn't just emotional relief — it can be a biological reset. At this stage of life, authenticity isn't optional if you want lasting health and vitality. It's not just a mindset shift; it can be the foundation for living a long, strong, and well life.

And here's the beauty: when your body feels safe, truth flows naturally. As energy steadies, you stop trying to perform authenticity and start embodying it. You can feel it — in the openness of your breath, the steadiness in your tone, the groundedness in your posture. Authenticity becomes less about effort and more about coherence — your biology and truth moving in rhythm.

For years, I tuned myself to everyone else's needs — changing my tone, my pace, my priorities to create harmony around me. But the moment I began tuning my life to my own truth, the noise faded. What remained was a clear, resonant signal that didn't waver under pressure. I stopped contorting myself to keep the peace and discovered that authenticity has its own frequency — strong enough to steady the entire room without forcing a thing.

Authenticity doesn't mean doing more; it means doing what's *real*. It's the quiet practice of allowing your truth to match your actions, your body to match your words. And when you do, your system recognizes it: your chest softens, your energy organizes itself, and something inside finally relaxes.

That's the heart of authenticity — not a performance, but a presence. The truth of who you are, lived out loud and felt all the way through.

When you live close to your truth, the body can hum with steadiness. When you override it, the current may flicker — not in one dramatic collapse, but in small moments: the yes that meant no, the silence that swallowed a need, the *fine* that wasn't.

That's where we'll go next — into the subtle ways disconnection begins, and how to find your way back.

The Cost of Self-Betrayal

Self-betrayal rarely arrives with a warning siren. It slips in quietly through choices that seem harmless: taking on one more task when you're stretched thin, dismissing a needed boundary, shelving a dream because wanting more feels selfish.

At first, each act feels small. But like pebbles in your shoe, they build with every step — rubbing blisters, altering your stride, and eventually leaving you limping. That's what years of self-betrayal do to the body — and the spirit.

I know this because I lived it. For years, I was known as the "Yes Woman." At work, I was the one who always delivered — no matter how tight the deadline. At home, I was the one who picked up the slack, volunteered, and made sure everything ran smoothly. On the surface, I looked strong and dependable. Inside, I was running on empty.

Each 'yes' I gave to others was a quiet 'no' to myself. And

the body keeps score. My sleep lessened, mornings were foggy, and my mood swung between wired and tired. At first, I brushed it off — stress, hormones, life. But the whispers grew louder: headaches that lingered, a body that couldn't rest, a mind that wouldn't quiet.

Your body can read every small self-betrayal as a stress signal — a quickened pulse, a subtle tightening, a shift in blood sugar or breath. And in midlife, when hormones may no longer cushion the stress response, each betrayal can feel more profound. What once felt manageable at thirty now can hit harder — not because resilience is fading, but because your body is finally done being ignored.

I remember the first time it happened — nothing was wrong, yet everything in me snapped. Out of nowhere, a wave of irritability ran through my body, sharp and sudden. There was no argument, no stressor, no reason — just a sudden surge, as if my system had hit capacity.

It wasn't a mood; it was a message. My body wasn't overreacting — it was overflowing. All the quiet yeses, the swallowed words, the skipped pauses had built until they spilled over. That moment wasn't failure — it was feedback. The body always speaks; midlife just turns up the volume.

This is why many women describe midlife as "falling apart." It isn't failure or age — it's a recall notice from your own system: *Please return to truth.*

One woman told me she couldn't remember the last time she'd gone a full day without saying yes to something she didn't want. By midlife, her body had become a map of exhaustion —

hormonal shifts, headaches, restless sleep, and fog that dull her edges. On paper, it looked like minor inconveniences. But beneath the surface lived years of energy poured into obligations that no longer matched her truth.

Self-betrayal can be expensive. It can rob vitality, drain clarity, and keep the body in a state of quiet survival mode. The world may applaud you for being dependable, agreeable, selfless — but your biology never misses the cost.

The encouraging part is that healing often begins the moment you start honoring yourself. Even one small act of authenticity may signal to your body that safety is possible. The nervous system can soften, stress may ease, and energy that once leaked through performance might begin to return. Each truthful choice becomes an opening — a gentle reminder that alignment is available, right here, right now.

Alignment often starts this way — not with grand gestures, but with a single reconciliation between what you feel and what you allow. And that's when the current can turn back on.

————————— *Turning Truth Into Power* —————————

If *living true* is the practice, truth is the pulse that keeps it alive. Here's the paradox: the very thing many of us were taught to soften, shrink, or hide — our truth — is often where our real power lives.

Something begins to shift each time that truth rises — whether whispered to yourself or shared with someone you trust. The body recognizes it before the mind does. The pulse steadies. The tension that once hummed beneath the skin begins to ease. What felt heavy starts to move again, as if energy once trapped in silence finally finds a way to flow.

Truth has a frequency — and when you speak it, every cell in your body tunes itself to that note. The dissonance between who you are and what you show starts to dissolve. What follows isn't drama or fireworks, but a deep, unmistakable exhale — the kind of relief that tells you your body has stopped bracing and started trusting again.

This isn't just relief. It's recalibration — your body remembering what alignment feels like.

The first time you say no without guilt, it can feel like setting down a weight you didn't realize you were carrying. The first time you stop explaining yourself, you notice how much energy returns. The first time you clearly name what you need, your body begins to trust you again — not just as a mind in motion, but as a place of care and truth.

Truth doesn't drain your energy — it restores it. That restoration is your aligned self re-emerging. It's like turning the power back on after a long blackout: the lights hum, the current returns, and suddenly everything feels alive again. With each practice — each honest word, each clear no, each quiet yes to yourself — the circuit grows stronger.

I still remember the first time I looked someone in the eye and said, "No, I can't take that on," without apology or explanation. It was such a small moment — one request, one boundary — yet it gave me back an entire evening, a full night's rest, and the quiet relief of waking without resentment in my body.

That's the thing about authenticity: it isn't performance or polish. It's what remains when the noise settles and truth is allowed to lead. The more you live from that place, the more natural it becomes — until one day you look back and realize this is who you've been all along. The rest was simply conditioning — learned over time, now ready to be gently unlearned.

This is the quiet math of midlife: Truth renews energy. Authenticity doesn't just free you — it fuels you. It becomes a steady current, carrying you into this next season with clarity, vitality, and a deeper sense of self-trust.

Because the truth — your truth — was never the problem. It was always the power.

The Quiet Magnetism of Truth

When you live in truth, something subtle yet powerful begins to shift. People feel it. They may not know what changed, but they sense it in your presence — the steadiness in your tone, the calm behind your eyes, in the way your energy no longer scatters.

You stop pushing to be seen. You stop chasing to be chosen. Instead, you take your place in the world with quiet certainty — and life begins to move toward you.

For years, I lived like a spotlight — swivelling toward others, trying to illuminate everything but myself. Until one day, I realized: light can guide without chasing. It doesn't apologize for the space it takes up. It simply stands steady, anchored in truth — my truth.

That was the turning point — the moment I stopped performing and started radiating.

That's what authenticity does — it gathers your energy back home. All the effort once spent proving, explaining, and pleasing returns to its source. Your nervous system settles into coherence. Your clarity deepens. And from that steadiness, magnetism naturally rises.

Truth creates resonance. It's not a force you project. It's a frequency you embody. People attuned to that frequency will find you. The ones who can't —won't. And that, too, is freedom.

Think of it like a lighthouse. It doesn't swivel to prove its worth or chase attention. It simply stands, unwavering and bright, guiding what's meant to find it. That's the quiet magnetism of truth — unforced, grounded, radiant.

Those were the leaks before — every yes I didn't mean, every forced smile, every late-night push that left me hollow. Each one a small betrayal that drained my light, like running on fumes with nothing left in the tank. But when authenticity replaced performance, the leaks sealed. My vitality no longer dripped away; it gathered, strengthened, and began to flow again.

Think of it like a faucet. When it leaks, gallons disappear unnoticed. But seal the leak, and suddenly that same water builds pressure, power, and flow. Your energy works the same way. When you stop apologizing for what's true, your vitality amplifies — not by force, but by integrity.

And here's the ripple effect: when you live aligned, your kids feel your calm, your partner notices your steadiness, and your colleagues trust your clarity. You don't have to push or persuade

— your presence becomes the permission slip they didn't know they were waiting for.

Authenticity doesn't shrink your influence — it expands it. When you live from truth, you stop leaking energy into performance and start radiating it into everything you touch.

The world often teaches women to become spotlights — to work harder, shine brighter, do more. But the truth invites something else entirely: stillness that signals strength. Presence that speaks without words.

And here's the paradox — the less you try to attract, the more aligned your world becomes. Because when you're anchored in truth, you stop chasing and start receiving. Energy that once scattered into performance now flows through coherence — a calm, consistent current.

When truth anchors you, you become magnetic by nature. This is the quiet power of living true: you no longer burn out to belong. You simply move with the energy that's been waiting to flow through you.

Embodied authenticity unlocks your power. And there's one more piece that ensures that power flows everywhere it needs to — that's where we'll go next.

TRY THIS: ONE SMALL TRUTH

At the end of today, pause and ask: *Where was I most authentic today?*

Note one moment—a clear no, a quiet truth, or a time you didn't shrink in a conversation.

Then ask: *How did my body respond?* Notice if your breath eased, if your shoulders softened, if energy returned?

That single truth isn't small; it's proof your system recognizes alignment — and rewards it immediately. Authenticity is like oxygen — it fills your system with truth. But oxygen on its own can dissipate. In the next chapter, we'll explore integrity, the current that keeps authenticity flowing through every part of your life. This is where integrity changes everything. Integrity isn't about perfection — it's about congruence. Each time your choices align with what you believe to be true, something seals.

CHAPTER 6

Integrity as an Energy Source

If authenticity asks, "Am I being true to myself right now?", integrity asks a different but equally important question: "Do my actions consistently line up with what I know to be true?"

Authenticity is the spark — the relief of dropping the mask, the breath of oxygen when you stop performing. Integrity is what can carry that spark forward. It's the current that can flow through your choices, your boundaries, and your commitments.

With authenticity, breath can find its rhythm. With integrity, that rhythm begins to move — quietly at first, then with power.

—— *Integrity: The Flow That Keeps You Alive* ——

If authenticity is breath, integrity can be the gentle current that lets it circulate through your life. Oxygen alone won't sustain you unless it circulates; in the same way, authenticity can fade unless integrity carries it into daily choices.

I learned this slowly — in the quiet consequences of good intentions that pulled me away from what mattered most. My family had planned a weekend getaway — a chance to relax, unplug, and reconnect. At the last minute, I stayed behind to finish a deadline. I told myself it was the "right thing to do," that it proved I was dependable and disciplined. But by the time I joined them, half the weekend was gone. My body was drained from late nights, and my mind was still spinning with unfinished tasks. I was physically there but emotionally absent — carrying guilt instead of joy, a soft heaviness beneath everything. Not sharp, but heavy, like a quiet ache reminding me how easily I drifted from what matters most.

That's what a blocked current can feel like — everything looks fine on the surface, but underneath, something has stopped moving. Each time I said yes when I meant no, or pushed past the whisper for rest, I could feel the flow tighten a little more. Even after the weekend ended, a quiet heaviness lingered — not just fatigue, but the knowing that I'd gone against myself.

Integrity moves like a river. When it runs clear, energy glides. Decisions clarify. Breath deepens. Stress can soften. But when it's dammed—by false yeses, over-explaining, or hiding what's true—the current shifts. The body often notices: the heart quickens, sleep lightens, the edges of calm fray. Energy leaks in many quiet ways. Each time your yes and no match, your body recharges.

And here's the beauty — integrity can clear the channel. Each time your truth is honored — whether that means saying no, resting when you're tired, or speaking what you really feel — you remove a branch from the river. Your breath moves deeper. Your nervous system steadies. A quiet warmth replaces tension. The current gathers strength again.

Integrity isn't a standard of perfection — it's the practice of living in sync with what you believe. It's about what you know is true with how you actually live. And when you do, your body recognizes it instantly. Instead of wasting energy on inner conflict, you reclaim it for a life of purpose. Integrity doesn't just guide your choices; it restores the life force you need to live them fully.

When "Doing the Right Thing" Isn't the Right Thing

You can follow every rule and still feel quietly emptied.

For years, I confused integrity with being 'good'. I thought it meant being reliable, responsible, and kind — even when it meant overriding my own needs. I showed up. I followed through. I said yes. And from the outside, it looked noble. It looked strong. It even looked like love.

But inside, it could feel like erosion.

Every time I swallowed what I needed to say, another small layer of energy slipped away. Each well-intentioned yes became a slow withdrawal from my own account. And even though it earned approval, It cost me something far more precious — my aliveness.

What finally landed was simple but radical: Integrity isn't

about being 'good'. It's about being **whole**.

And integrity is not morality — it's energetic.

Notice what softens in your body as that truth lands.

I remember the moment this finally came into focus. A friend had invited me to a small dinner — nothing fancy, just good food, connection, and a chance to exhale. I wanted to go. My body wanted to go. But at the last minute, I convinced myself I should stay home and squeeze in more work.

By the time I arrived, the meal was half over. The room was warm with laughter and easy conversation, the kind you can feel in your bones. And there I was — stepping in with a tight chest, stressed and wired from the day, struggling to shift gears, struggling to relax. Everyone else was present; I was still catching up to myself.

That's when it landed: this wasn't about being responsible. It was an energy leak — the cost of choosing the version of me I thought people expected over the truth that was asking to be honored.

Energy leaks rarely vanish on their own; they can collect — in the background noise of unmet needs and postponed truths. One small compromise at a time, the current thins. Your vitality softens. What once fueled you now flickers, not because you're aging, but because you're out of alignment.

Your body isn't broken; it may be whispering: *Stop the leak. Come home.*

Think of it as an energy account you've been drawing from for years. At first, the balance seems endless. But over time, each withdrawal — each self-abandonment masked as doing "the right thing" — adds up. Eventually, the account dips low, and your body sends the bill.

It's the kind of truth that asks for a slow breath before it settles. Let that breath loosen whatever tightened as you read these words.

Instead of repairing tissues or balancing hormones, your body reroutes its reserves to manage the constant crisis of misalignment.

The result can be hot flashes that wake you, cravings that tug you off track, and moods that rise like waves you can't predict.

This isn't failure. It's a flare. Your body's way of saying, *I'm overdrawn.*

Integrity in midlife may be less about handling more and more about honoring what's been whispering for years.

Every small act of realignment — resting instead of pushing, speaking instead of swallowing, saying no instead of defaulting to yes — is a deposit. Little by little, you stop draining and start refueling.

Alignment becomes less about discipline and more about devotion — a quiet rhythm that replenishes you from the inside out. It's the shift from running on fumes to running on flow. The kind that carries you, steady and whole, into everything that comes next.

Integrity as the Power Grid

Think of integrity as your personal power grid.

When your thoughts, words, and actions line up, energy flows cleanly. You think, *I need more rest.* You tell your family, *I'm heading to bed early tonight.* And you actually turn out the lights at ten. The current hums. You wake clearer, lighter, and — most importantly — you've kept the promise you made to yourself.

But when they don't line up, the system shorts out. You think, *I'm exhausted,* but you say, *Sure, I'll finish this project tonight and* then stay up scrolling past midnight. Your body may register that misfire — you might wake feeling drained, edgy, already behind before the day begins. Another fuse blown. Another circuit strained.

Integrity isn't tested in the big moments. It's built — or drained — in the small, ordinary choices you make each day. Each override dims your internal light just a little more. The current weakens right when you need it most.

That's why many women say they wake up exhausted — even after a full night of sleep — or feel spent by noon without any apparent reason. It's not weakness. It's not lack of discipline. It's the quiet cost of living out of integrity — running on a patchwork of half-truths and *shoulds* while your body pays the bill.

I began to see it clearly in my own life. My family has always been my top priority — my heart, my anchor, my why. But my choices didn't always reflect that. Work often won, disguised as responsibility. On paper, it looked like devotion. In truth, it was another blown fuse — a mismatch between what I valued most and how I was actually showing up.

My health carried the fallout. The late nights, the endless striving, the quiet guilt of not being fully present — it all registered in my body. Exhaustion that lingered no matter how much I slept. Weight that refused to shift. A nervous system humming on high alert.

My energy wasn't just dipping; it was unraveling. Misalignment can short the current of your *Aligned Identity* — and the moment integrity returns, your system hums again. Because misalignment doesn't just drain you emotionally — it taxes your biology.

Midlife became my turning point. What I once saw as my body betraying me, I now recognize as an invitation — a natural pause that asked me to rewire my life. It forced me to stop running on the old operating system, the one powered by proving and pushing. It asked me to build a cleaner current — one where my choices finally reflected my true priorities, and my physiology could trust me again.

Integrity isn't about getting it all right. It's about being consistent with what's right for you. And each small act of congruence is like flipping breakers back on. One by one, the rooms of your inner house light up again.

Here's the more profound truth: integrity isn't restriction — it's restoration. Each act of congruence repairs your internal circuitry, creating a steadiness that becomes renewable energy — not a surge, but a rhythm you can lean into. And the beautiful part? That steadiness becomes magnetic. People notice themselves softening around you. They adjust without knowing why. Because when you move from coherence, it quietly invites others into balance.

That's why integrity isn't a moral ideal — it's your power grid. And when you repair the wiring, energy returns — not in bursts, but in a calm, steady current that sustains you for the long haul.

— *When Your Body Sends the Bill* —

The truth about misalignment is that it's felt long before it's seen. You can override your truth for a while — push through, explain it away — but your body keeps quiet record. And eventually, the bill can come due.

It looks like this:
- You promise yourself you'll rest, but then you scroll through your phone until midnight. *Receipt.*
- You commit to eating lighter, then reach for takeout because you're too drained to cook. *Receipt.*
- You tell a friend, "It's no problem," while quietly resenting the extra load. *Receipt.*

Each of those moments may seem small, but together they drain your reserves — one micro-leak at a time. A knot in your stomach. A fog that lingers behind your eyes. Hot flashes that flare harder when you're stretched too thin. These aren't random annoyances — they're *itemized charges* from your body, showing you exactly where you've been living out of integrity.

The difference now is that the costs come faster — and they ask to be paid in energy. As hormonal rhythms evolve, your stress buffer may thin. Your body becomes more responsive, more honest. Cortisol levels can spike more quickly; inflammation can linger longer. In practice, every false yes, every ignored boundary, every overextension costs more now than it once did.

It's not punishment. It's precision. Your body no longer lets you get away with what once slipped under the radar.

I often see this in women. One client told me she agreed to volunteer for a school fundraiser while also caring for her aging mother and managing a full-time job. She smiled and said yes, wanting to help. But by week's end, her sleep unraveled, her hot flashes intensified, and she snapped at her family over nothing. On paper, it was "just one more thing." But her body read it differently — another withdrawal from an account already in the red.

The truth is, borrowing against yourself can only go so long before it shows up in energy. The only way to stop the drain is to align your words, actions, and choices with what's *truly at your core* — the values you refuse to compromise, the identity that feels most aligned.

When those pieces click into place, the current steadies. Energy stops scattering and begins to gather. It strengthens, stabilizes, and flows toward the life you actually want to live.

Integrity isn't perfection — it's repair. And repair happens in the small things. Each honest no. Each boundary honored. Each moment you choose truth over convenience. Every micro-alignment is a payment made — not to guilt or obligation, but to your own vitality.

Over time, those small deposits rebuild trust — with your body, your energy, and your self-worth. That's the real wealth of integrity: a nervous system that knows you'll keep your word, and a body that finally feels safe to exhale.

———————— *Integrity Stops the Leaks* ————————

Energy doesn't only come from what you add — it comes from what you stop losing.

Think of integrity as plugging the leaks in your system. Every time you override your truth with a polite yes, push through when your body begs for rest, or bite your tongue to avoid conflict, a little energy drains away. At first, you barely notice. But over weeks and years, those leaks add up to exhaustion you can't explain.

Sometimes the leaks are subtle — walking on eggshells when you're afraid to speak your truth, tolerating behavior that makes you feel small, or letting someone disrespect you without saying a word. Other times, they're obvious — staying in environments that drain you, silencing your needs to keep the peace, or forcing yourself to show up as someone you're not. Every compromise can erode vitality.

This is where integrity changes everything. Integrity doesn't demand perfection; it calls you back to alignment. Each time your choices align with what you believe to be true, something seals — a small restoration inside. Your nervous system stops bracing. Your hormones stop overcompensating. Your body doesn't waste energy holding you in survival mode.

One woman in my group described it like patching holes in a bucket. "No matter how much water I poured in — workouts, supplements, vacations — I was still drained. The leaks were my false yeses and ignored boundaries. Once I started plugging those, the same amount of effort finally filled me up."

When integrity stops the leaks, your body has a chance to restore itself. And that's the foundation for the next shift: energy on demand.

Energy on Demand

When you live in integrity, you don't just feel lighter — you gain your power back. It's like plugging your body into a steady current after years of running on a flickering generator. Suddenly, the energy is clean, stable, and reliable. It moves through you without breakdowns or burnout.

One of my clients told me she couldn't remember the last time she woke without dread. Mornings felt like dragging a boulder uphill. Coffee cut through the fog just enough to start the day, but by mid-afternoon, she was crashing — reaching for sugar, scrolling for distraction, pushing through on empty. She kept telling herself she needed more discipline.

What changed everything wasn't more willpower — it was alignment. She began practicing integrity in the smallest ways: saying no when she meant it. Honoring her bedtime instead of answering one more email. Speaking up in meetings instead of staying silent to keep the peace.

Within weeks, something shifted — she began to notice the difference. One morning she told me,

"I woke before my alarm. For the first time in years, I didn't feel behind before the day even started. I felt like my body trusted me again."

That's the quiet magic of integrity. Each aligned act restores energy across your systems:

- Cortisol steadies; old surges soften into rhythm.
- Blood sugar finds balance as cravings release their grip.
- Sleep deepens; rest becomes a refuge again.
- Inflammation quiets; your body feels the safety it's been waiting for.

And with each breath, the current grows steadier.

Imagine waking tomorrow with every cell humming like quiet electricity. You sip your coffee not to survive, but to savor. You move through the day making choices that feel clean, clear, and congruent.

This can become a kin of energy on demand. Not the kind you chase — the kind you cultivate. It doesn't come from pushing harder or doing more. It flows naturally when your truth and your actions finally match.

That's the unspoken formula of integrity: each aligned choice amplifies energy across your systems — until what once felt like effort becomes your new ease.

———— *When Truth and Body Move as One* ————

When you live in integrity, your body doesn't just stop leaking energy — it starts radiating it. Alignment isn't passive repair; it's an active current that lifts you higher than you thought possible.

When your actions align with your truth, you move through life with a steadier sense of purpose. That's the current of your *aligned self* — embodied integrity in motion. You have energy for what excites you, clarity for what matters, and resilience to follow through. Creativity flows more freely, problem-solving feels natural, and you meet challenges with objectivity instead of depletion.

But the shift runs deeper than energy. When you live from the vibration of integrity, you begin to *resonate* — your presence changes. There's a grounded calm in your eyes, a steadiness people can feel before you say a word. And from that steadiness, doors open. Opportunities can appear — not because you chase them, but because you've become magnetic to what matches your frequency.

Happiness stops being something to chase. It becomes the state from which you operate. A quiet excitement fuels your days — not in rare bursts, but as a rhythm your body recognizes as home.

Living authentically with integrity isn't just a path to health. It's the foundation for expansion — a way of moving through the world that restores vitality, amplifies presence, and lets joy take up residence where stress once lived.

When truth and body move as one, energy can feel less like something you chase and more like something you embody.

TRY THIS: ONE KEPT PROMISE

For the next three days, choose one small promise to yourself — and honor it.

It doesn't have to be grand. It could be closing the laptop when you said you would. Speaking up when something crosses your line. Or honoring a boundary with food, rest, or screen time.

At the end of each day, pause gently and ask yourself:
- Did I keep **that promise?**
- If yes, how did my body respond? (Notice steadiness, ease, or a little more energy in **your system.**)
- If not, what got in the way — and what would integrity have looked **like instead?**

As you repeat this for three days, you'll start to see something subtle but powerful. Integrity isn't a single moment — it's a rhythm. Each micro-agreement you keep becomes a quiet message to your body: *you can trust me.*

With every kept promise, your energy steadies.

Your nervous system unclenches.

Your sense of power grows — not from control, but from congruence.

This is integrity in real time: not abstract, not distant, but a shift you can *feel.* Practice it through small, doable choices, and over time your body learns that alignment is safe — and energy flows back in naturally.

With authenticity and integrity, you now have the foundation: **oxygen and current.**

In Part 2, we'll add the compass — your **values** — so the energy you've reclaimed can finally guide you where you're meant to go.

PART ONE

INTEGRATION EXERCISE

The Alignment Reset

This is where you stop thinking about authenticity and integrity — and start feeling them in your body. Do this daily, and watch how it rewires not just your choices, but your biology.

Step 1. Name the Leak
Close your eyes and scan your day. Where did you negotiate against yourself? A false yes, a swallowed truth, a moment you pushed when you needed rest. Don't judge it — just notice. Whisper to yourself: *"That was a leak."* Awareness begins the repair.

Step 2. Place a Hand on Your Body
Bring one hand to your chest, the other to your belly. Feel your breath move beneath your palms. This simple touch tells your nervous system: *I'm here. I'm listening.*

Step 3. Ask the Integrity Question
Quietly ask: *"What would be the most honest move right now?"* Don't analyze. Let your body answer — a word, an image, a sensation. The truthful option often feels lighter, clearer, or

more grounded. That whisper is your *aligned self* speaking —
listen before logic takes over.

Step 4. Anchor in Truth

Take one slow breath and whisper: *Today, I stop negotiating
with myself.* Notice what shifts — the softening in your shoulders, the lengthening of your spine, the widening of your ribs.
That's your biology aligning with your truth.

Step 5. Seal It With a Micro-Action

Choose one tiny action in the next 60 seconds that reflects what
you just felt. Send the text. Close the laptop. Pour the water. Say
no kindly. Integrity doesn't wait — it's practiced in real time.
Each micro-alignment teaches your body: truth is safe.

Step 6. Celebrate the Shift

Pause and feel the after-state. Is your breath deeper? Shoulders
looser? Mind clearer? This is your body saying *thank you*.
These micro-wins aren't small — they're rewiring your nervous
system to live in alignment.

Integration Note:

You don't need hours. This can take less than five minutes.
Done daily, it moves authenticity and integrity from ideas into
embodied strength — a renewable energy source you can trust.
Each time you pause, breathe, and act from truth, you rewire
your body to trust you again. That trust is energy you can
carry forward.

2

Part Two

Living By Your Core Values

CHAPTER 7

The Compass Within

With authenticity and integrity anchoring you, values become your navigation system — the map that keeps truth moving in the right direction.

What Values Really Are

Take a slow breath and notice what steadies you when life feels noisy. That calm awareness is where your values live—before words, before thought.

Before we dive in, let's get clear on what I mean by values.

Values aren't slogans or vision-board words. They're the quiet principles that tend to steer your choices all day long—whether you notice them or not.

Think of values as your inner compass. They don't measure speed; they point to true north. When you live more in sync with them, life can feel lighter and clearer.

When you drift, stress often builds, symptoms speak up, and

your body lets you know something's off.

Some values shift with seasons—adventure in your 20s, stability in your 40s. Others feel like non-negotiables: cross them and your energy drains, your peace frays. Name the non-negotiables and drifting begins to slow.

Pause for a moment and sense this in your own body. If you're unsure whether a value is real, notice how your body responds: truth feels steady, borrowed values feel tight.

Values set direction; non-negotiables add guardrails. Together, they offer compass and protection.

—— *Why Values Matter More Than Willpower* ——

Many of us were taught that discipline is the answer. Try harder. Push longer. Stick to the plan. However, willpower tends to fade—especially under stress or fatigue. Values are different. They don't rely on force; they provide direction.

You can feel the difference. Willpower tightens the jaw; values relax the breath. They're more likely to hold when motivation runs low.

When daily choices line up with your values, decisions feel lighter and less draining. When they don't, your body flags the cost. Stress hormones rise, energy dips. Symptoms like restless sleep, brain fog, or anxiety can grow louder.

For many women, midlife magnifies misalignment. Shifts in this season have a way of turning up the volume on what's not working. The answer isn't more effort; it's alignment. Willpower burns out. Your compass doesn't.

But knowing that and living it can be two very different things.

Living by Shoulds

I'll be honest with you. I drifted so far out of alignment with my values that I no longer knew what they were.

I lived by expectations—what I "should" do, how I "should" act, what I "should" prioritize. From the outside, I looked reliable. Inside, I felt hollow. I said yes when I meant no. Over-committed until my body ached, smiled when I wanted to set a boundary. Reliable on paper; invisible to myself.

When I finally looked inward, it hit hard: I'd been running on borrowed values. The unlearning took time—weeks, then months—peeling back conditioning, facing where I'd betrayed myself, asking: What truly matters? What am I no longer willing to carry? If I put truth first, who might I disappoint?

It was one of the toughest exercises I've done—and one of the most rewarding. Because once I uncovered my values—not the ones I thought I should have, but the ones that made me feel alive—it felt like I'd been handed a compass I didn't know I was missing. Decisions grew clearer. My yes and no meant something. Alignment wasn't just a mindset—it was energy, direction, and a felt sense of freedom.

What surprised me most: the moment I began to realign with my actual values, clarity followed. Second-guessing eased.

My body settled. My mind quieted. Peace didn't have to be

chased—it tended to arrive when I stopped betraying myself.

That's the gift of values: they strip away the noise so you can hear your aligned self again. Without that compass, life becomes reactive. You're pulled by currents—other people's needs, outside expectations, the endless list of "shoulds." One day you're paddling hard in one direction, the next you're spun around to another. It's exhausting, not because you're weak, but because there's no true north to guide you.

And that's the real cost of drifting: your nervous system rarely gets to rest, your body burns energy it doesn't have, and midlife signals can grow louder with every wave. When you reconnect with your values, it's like finally seeing the lighthouse through the fog. You choose your course with clarity, conserve energy, and feel steadier even when the waters are rough.

That's why values matter. If you don't know them, you'll keep reacting instead of steering. When you do, everything starts to align.

Lost Without a Map

There's little more unsettling than moving fast in the wrong direction. Pause for a second and notice how your shoulders respond when you read the word "unsettling." That tightening is what life without direction feels like.

I know this feeling well. "For years I took pride in being driven and disciplined. I was always going somewhere—but if I'm honest, I wasn't sure where "there" even was.

That's what life without values can feel like: constant motion without direction. You can have energy, ambition, and even success, but without a compass, you drift. You end up drained, frustrated, and quietly wondering why all the effort doesn't feel more fulfilling.

I'll never forget when this hit hardest. I was saying yes to everything—projects, social commitments, responsibilities—because I thought that's what a "capable" woman did. My calendar was packed, my to-do list never ended, and people praised how much I could juggle.

But inside, I was unraveling. Exhausted, snappy with the people I loved, lying awake at night thinking, "Why am I working this hard if I don't even feel good?" I realized I wasn't living my life—I was living by everyone else's expectations.

- That's what happens when you don't know your values. You let the loudest voice in the room set your direction. You let external applause drown out internal truth.

- Most of us aren't lost because we lack willpower. We're lost because we never paused to chart what matters most. When you don't know your true north, you rely on guesswork, outside voices, or ingrained habits that were never truly yours.

- Values are that compass. They don't tell you how fast to move—they tell you where to go.

When Alignment Changes Everything

By the time we reach midlife, the cracks are harder to gloss over. Years of saying yes when we meant no, of swallowing truth to keep the peace, of pushing our needs aside—each choice accumulates. And every compromise chips away at self-trust.

Every time you silence your voice, you reinforce the lie that your needs don't matter. Over time, that erosion doesn't just leave you tired—it can leave you feeling invisible to yourself. That's the deeper cost of drifting: not just stress or exhaustion, but the quiet ache that whispers, "I don't even know who I am anymore." It rarely happens all at once. It's subtle—one ignored boundary, one false yes, one borrowed role at a time. One day, you realize you've built a life around values that were never truly yours.

Midlife has a way of stripping away the ability to outrun it. The body won't hold that tension forever. Relationships struggle on half-truths. And your sense of self only stays buried for so long.

Alignment matters because the cost of drifting isn't just exhaustion—it's losing your connection to yourself, to the people you love, and to the life you're meant to live.

The Badge of Dependability

One client wore dependability like a badge of honor. She was the woman everyone counted on—the one who never said no, who carried the weight for everyone else. On the surface, it appeared to be loyalty and strength.

Underneath, she was running on fumes. Her real values were health and family, yet her choices betrayed them daily — pushing through exhaustion, skipping rest, giving her loved one's leftovers.

When she realigned, the change was undeniable. She said no to what drained her. She treated rest as sacred, not selfish.

Very quickly, her family felt the difference. Her kids got her laughter back. Her partner got warmth instead of irritation.

She stopped feeling invisible and started feeling powerful— not because she did more, but because she finally lived true.

She learned that saying no wasn't neglect—it was nourishment. As she honored rest as non-negotiable, her body softened, her laughter returned, and her home filled with ease again.

The Mother of Five

Another client, a devoted mother of five, believed that being a "good mom" meant being available every second. Every ride, every crisis, every late-night request—she answered them all.

She believed sacrifice was the price of love. Over time, her health buckled under the weight. Anxiety, sleepless nights, and frayed patience became her norm.

Her deepest value was presence—yet her choices stole the very connection she longed for. When she realigned, her home shifted. She created rhythms of rest. She learned to say no without guilt.

And her kids noticed. Instead of snapping, she listened. Instead of showing up exhausted, she showed up calm. They no longer got her scraps—they got her presence. Honoring her values wasn't selfish. It was the most loving thing she could do.

The Power Struggle Marriage

I've also seen alignment transform marriages. One woman shared how every conflict with her husband turned into a stand-off. Each dug in, clinging to the need to be right. Arguments dragged on, unresolved, leaving them cold and disconnected.

Then she uncovered her core values: respect, love, and truth. For the first time, she filtered her reactions through them. Instead of defending her ego, she asked, "What response honors respect? What action reflects love?" That shift changed everything.

Arguments gave way to conversations; winning gave way to understanding. Respect returned. Intimacy grew. Alignment didn't just change her—it changed her marriage.

What shifts in our lives is mirrored in our bodies. This is the inner power of values. They're not just abstract principles—they're the compass that steadies your body, heals relationships, and frees energy. When you drift from them, life unravels.

When you realign, you stop burning out, stop fighting yourself, and begin living with the clarity, peace, and strength that were waiting inside you all along. These stories show alignment in real life—and they point to something deeper: alignment isn't just emotional; it's biological.

Your body keeps score of whether you're living in sync with your values. When you honor your truth, your nervous system eases, stress hormones settle, and energy flows toward repair and vitality. When you betray it, cortisol spikes, muscles tense, and inflammation can rise.

Over time, the difference shows up not just in how you feel, but in how your body functions. Alignment is physiology in action.

Alignment Lives in the Body

Alignment isn't just a mindset. It's a physiological state—one your body recognizes long before your mind catches up.

You've felt it: the deep exhale when something feels right, the quiet calm after you finally tell the truth, the lightness in your chest when your actions match your inner knowing.

That's alignment—biology in motion.

Here's the part many women miss: You can know your values intellectually and still struggle to live them if your body is out of balance.

If your nervous system is fried, you may default to people-pleasing just to avoid conflict. If your hormones are swinging, mood shifts can hijack clarity. If your gut is inflamed, anxiety can drown out your inner compass.

This is why so many women in midlife feel stuck.

It's not that you don't know what matters—it's that your body may be too depleted or dysregulated to follow through. Values may light the way, but without steadiness, energy, and resilience, even the clearest compass is hard to honor.

When you live in sync with your values, your nervous system recognizes safety. Stress hormones settle. Muscles unclench. Energy that once went into defense flows back toward repair, digestion, and renewal. Sleep deepens. Focus sharpens. Cravings quiet.

It's not magic—it's physiology responding to congruence. And your body will also tell you when you've drifted. Say yes when you mean no, and your pulse quickens. Swallow your truth, and your breath shortens. Ignore your needs, and your system shifts toward emergency mode—cortisol spikes, inflammation rises, and energy drains faster than you can refill it.

Over time, that chemistry writes a story in your tissues: fatigue, tension, restless sleep, a hum of unease. Your body isn't betraying you—it's protecting you. It's the messenger, not the mistake.

Every symptom is feedback about whether you're living from truth or from habit. When you honor your values, your body answers back. Your breath deepens. Your shoulders drop. Peace doesn't have to be chased—it becomes a physiological response to alignment.

Identity + values + biology — that's the trifecta of alignment.

Identity offers consistency. Values give direction. Biology gives fuel. Together, they make alignment not just possible, but sustainable. Because naming your values is only the beginning. The real transformation comes when you live them—especially when life tests you, tempts you, or pressures you to drift.

When your body feels safe, truth flows more naturally. And when you live aligned, you stop burning out.

Alignment doesn't live only in thoughts. It lives in breath, pulse, and choices. It's the quiet intelligence that whispers, this is right for me.

And that's the moment things change—when your biology, your values, and your identity finally move in the same direction.

Meeting Your Compass

Feel your feet on the ground, as if standing there now—earth solid beneath you, air moving around you.

Imagine yourself at a crossroads. Roads stretch in every direction. Some look tempting, some familiar, some easy. Without a guide, you'd stand there second-guessing every step.

Now imagine a compass in your hand. Its needle points steadily toward your true north—the values that matter most. As you watch it settle, your shoulders drop. You exhale. You realize you don't have to figure everything out or chase every shiny distraction. You follow the needle.

This is what it can feel like to live by your values. The anxiety of guessing eases. The tension of overthinking softens. You don't waste energy debating every choice, because alignment brings peace.

I know this because I've lived the other side. For years, I wasn't just detached from my values—I was detached from myself. The hollowness I described was the cost of drifting too far.

My body reflected that distance—like carrying a compass that spun aimlessly while a rubber band inside me wound tighter and tighter. No matter how much I achieved or pushed, the tension didn't ease, because I wasn't guided by what truly mattered.

Coming home to my values was liberating. It's why this book exists. When I uncovered what truly mattered—not the roles I thought I had to fill, not absorbed expectations, but the deep, personal truths that lit me up—the rubber band loosened. My body relaxed. My energy steadied. I felt like I was finally living my life, not someone else's version of it.

When I named my core values, the shift was profound. One of the clearest for me was health. And here's the irony: everyone around me thought health was already who I was—I worked out, ate whole foods, looked the part.

But I was betraying that value every time I said yes when I needed rest, every time I pushed through exhaustion instead of honoring recovery, every time I lived by expectation instead of authenticity.

That quiet misalignment cost more than any skipped workout. Once I claimed health as a core value—not just something I did, but something I lived from—everything simplified. Sleep became sacred. Boundaries felt natural. Energy steadied because my choices no longer betrayed what mattered most.

For me, it was health. For you, it might be family, freedom, creativity, or something else. The compass looks different for each of us, but the effect is similar: when you live in alignment with your values, your body notices—and responds. In steadier energy. In deeper rest. In the quiet confidence of living from the inside out.

——————— *Naming Your Values* ———————

Most of us have never been asked to clearly name our values. We inherit them—family, culture, religion, work. We end up living by "shoulds" instead of truths. By midlife, the weight of roles can make it hard to discern which values are truly ours and which were borrowed.

That's why identifying your values matters. Once you uncover your own—not the ones imposed on you—you may feel like you've been handed a missing compass. Decisions feel lighter. Choices stop being tug-of-wars. You finally recognize the feel of alignment.

Values don't usually appear just because you want them to. They reveal themselves in how you feel, in the patterns of your choices, and even in your body's signals. Think of them as buried stones—hidden under years of noise and conditioning. As you unearth them, each becomes a marker on your path.

Your body is often the first place hidden values surface. In alignment, your whole body exhales. Tension eases, posture relaxes, breath returns to a natural rhythm. It's the quiet relief of no longer bracing—a settling that says, "This fits."

Out of alignment, your body braces—muscles tighten, restlessness builds, inflammation takes hold. It's a built-in compass that hums when you're on track and screeches when you're off.

Joy is another clue. Recall moments when time disappeared—a belly laugh with a friend, a quiet walk in nature, losing yourself in a project. Those sparks aren't accidents; they're flares of truth showing which values are alive when you feel most yourself.

The opposite is just as revealing: the exhaustion after saying yes when you meant no, the resentment when boundaries are ignored, the bone-deep fatigue of autopilot. These are warning lights on your dashboard—not failures, but flags that a core value is being crossed.

Longing can also point the way. The "if only" thoughts—If only I had more time… If only I could stop…—aren't indulgent daydreams. They're breadcrumbs. Follow them and you'll uncover values waiting beneath duty and expectation.

And then there's vision. Picture yourself five years from now, not just surviving but thriving. What fills your days? Who's around you? How does your body feel as you move through that life? This isn't fantasy—it's your values showing where they want to lead you.

Over time, these signals—the body's whispers, sparks of joy, warning lights, longings, and a clear vision—begin to repeat. That repetition isn't random. It's your compass revealing itself, pointing you back to core truths that have been there all along.

My invitation: pay attention. Become the detective of your own body and life. Each clue is a breadcrumb leading you back to yourself. Follow them long enough, and you'll find alignment isn't something you manufacture—it's something you uncover.

For much of my life. I didn't realize how far I had drifted from what mattered. I couldn't have named my values if you asked." to "Without realizing it, I had drifted far from the things that once grounded me. If someone had asked me what I stood for, I'm not sure I could have answered.

When I finally named my values, I didn't just write words on a page—I uncovered myself. It was raw and sometimes painful, like peeling back years of "shoulds" and roles. But seeing those truths on paper felt like looking in a mirror and recognizing myself again.

From that moment, decisions grew clearer and less draining—because I wasn't guessing. I was rooted again, steady in who I was.

You don't need a perfect list. Start with three that feel alive in your body—you can refine as you live them.

Choosing Your Compass

The shift is simple and powerful: choose your values—or the world will likely choose for you.

When you consciously name what matters most, you take back authority. You stop drifting. You stop handing power to outside voices, cultural expectations, or constant urgency. You steer with steadiness instead of scrambling in reaction.

Think of values like guardrails on a winding road. They don't limit freedom—they protect it. Without guardrails, every curve feels risky. With them, you move with confidence, supported in staying the course.

Here's the quiet magic: when your values are clear, the noise inside tends to quiet.

Decisions that once felt heavy stop being battles. The inner tug-of-war that drains so much energy finally eases. You don't juggle a dozen competing "shoulds." You have a steady framework to recognize what belongs and what doesn't.

A client of mine built her career on being "the fixer." She stayed late, picked up slack, rescued every crisis—even when it wasn't hers. People admired her reliability, but inside she was unraveling. Her phone buzzed constantly, meals were rushed at her desk, evenings with family were interrupted by emails she felt she couldn't ignore.

She equated productivity with worth and gave her power to everyone else's emergencies. When she named her core values—peace, family, integrity—everything shifted. She realized constant rescuing wasn't integrity; it was self-abandonment.

She stopped answering every late-night email, protected family dinners, and let colleagues carry their own weight. For the first time in decades, she wasn't reacting to chaos—she was leading from her compass. The result? More respect at work, deeper connection at home, and a quiet confidence that comes from living her truth.

This is the moment many women describe as lightness. Not because life suddenly got easy, but because they stopped fighting themselves.

Every time you honor a value, you strengthen the muscle of integrity and your capacity to live with more energy and peace.

TRY THIS: FEEL YOUR COMPASS

Find a quiet spot and sit comfortably. Place one hand over your heart or your belly—whichever feels grounding.

- **Name a value**. Whisper one of your core values—health, love, freedom, honesty, or whatever feels true.

- **Notice your body.** As you hold that value in mind, pay attention: does your breath deepen? Do your shoulders soften? Do you feel a spark of energy or a sense of calm?

- **Shift to contrast.** Recall a recent moment when you drifted from that value—maybe saying yes when you meant no, or pushing when you needed rest. Notice your body's language—tightening, heaviness, restlessness, or another sensation.

- **Return home.** Come back to your value. Imagine carrying it into tomorrow and making one choice that honors it fully. Take a final breath. That's alignment—a felt signal you're on track.

Naming your values gives direction; living them requires boundaries—your non-negotiables.

CHAPTER 8

Naming the Non-Negotiables

In the last chapter, you uncovered your compass — the values that point you toward your true north. But direction alone isn't enough. To live aligned, you must also protect those values. That protection comes from non-negotiables — the clear lines that act as anchors, keeping your compass steady when life tests you.

The Power of the Line in the Sand

For years, my calendar looked like a badge of honor — back-to-back meetings, endless commitments, late-night projects, marathon training. From the outside, it seemed like I had mastered balance. Beneath the surface, I was stretched thin, restless, and quietly exhausted.

The truth was, I hadn't paused to decide what mattered most. Without that clarity, every request felt urgent, every opportunity necessary, every invitation an obligation. I mistook busyness for purpose — until my body exposed the truth.

What unraveled wasn't just time management; it was misalignment with my true self. Unknowingly, health was the first thing I bartered away — traded for someone else's urgency, for fear of missing out, for the pressure to keep proving I could handle it all. And my body kept every receipt: sleepless nights, simmering anxiety, and the kind of fatigue no green smoothie could fix.

Midlife only sharpened the message. The costs of ignoring myself became undeniable. It wasn't one symptom — it felt like living inside a storm where the weather shifted without warning. One moment clear and steady; the next, a swirl of fatigue, restlessness, and intensity. My body became the messenger I could no longer ignore.

I had been dismissing that messenger for years — pushing through late nights, meeting deadlines at two in the morning, then convincing myself I could still run a marathon on a few hours of sleep. On the outside: discipline. On the inside: self-neglect dressed up as achievement.

The breaking point came at the 32-kilometer mark of my marathon. My body gave out. I was rushed to the hospital and learned my heart markers were in a dangerous range and my blood glucose unstable. The alarm was loud enough to hear.

What haunts me most isn't the collapse itself — it's the horror my family felt hearing my name announced over the PA, not as a triumphant finisher but as an emergency. In that moment, my choices weren't just costing me; they were shaking the people I love.

That day, I stopped chasing strength and started cultivating stewardship. It was the wake-up call I couldn't outrun. Health was no longer something I admired from afar — it became a **non-negotiable**.

That decision didn't make life smaller. It made it clearer. The tug-of-war ended. Choices simplified because the line was already drawn.

That's the power of non-negotiables. They aren't walls to shut people out. They're anchors that hold you steady — in integrity, in alignment, in wholeness.

— *What Non-Negotiables Really Are (and Aren't)* —

Non-negotiables aren't restrictions. They're declarations.

They are the values and boundaries you choose not to trade — no matter how shiny the opportunity or how loud the pressure.

Think of them as the foundation of a house. Without them, the structure wobbles in every storm. With them, you can build higher and stronger, trusting the ground beneath you.

Many women resist naming non-negotiables for fear of appearing rigid, selfish, or difficult. In practice, the opposite tends to be true. Naming them doesn't make you selfish — it makes you trustworthy to yourself. Non-negotiables don't close doors — they open the right ones. They don't cut people off — they clarify which connections deserve your energy. They don't make you less available — they make you more present where it counts.

Here's the hidden gift: non-negotiables free you from decision fatigue. Once the line is drawn, you don't spend energy justifying, explaining, or wrestling with guilt. You already know, because the compass is set.

And in midlife, this clarity is more than a convenience — it can be a lifeline. With shifting energy and competing demands, every unnecessary yes drains the system. Every choice out of alignment compounds stress. Living by your non-negotiables creates safety and stability when other things feel uncertain.

I learned this the hard way. As a freelance statistician on a massive project, I pulled in two additional statisticians to meet crushing deadlines. One Friday I said, "All hands on deck this weekend." One of them looked me in the eye: "That won't happen. I don't work weekends or evenings. At 5 p.m. Friday, I shut down and I'm back at 9 a.m. Monday."

My jaw dropped. I thought, What nerve! How selfish.

It took years — and a round of burnout — to see she had it right. She valued health, rest, and life outside work — and protected those values with non-negotiables. Meanwhile, I was flushing mine away. She left work restored; I left drained. Boundaries weren't about being difficult. They were about being whole. Non-negotiables weren't selfish. They were survival.

The Cost of Blurred Lines

When you don't name your non-negotiables, you become a magnet for misalignment.

People sense they can push your edges, so they do. Overload follows. Resentment builds. Life starts to feel like it belongs to everyone but you.

The body feels it, too. Stress hormones surge when you keep saying yes against your will. Cortisol ramps up; cravings and weight changes can follow. Inflammation creeps in when rest and recovery get sacrificed. Sleep suffers because your nervous system never gets the signal that it's safe to shut down.

Emotionally, the toll is steep. Each broken promise to yourself chips away at self-trust. Doubt grows. Guilt creeps in. Confidence erodes. You stop feeling like the driver and more like a passenger being dragged along.

This is why many women in midlife describe feeling un-recognizable to themselves. It's not only shifting biology. It's years of fuzzy boundaries, compromise stacked on compromise until the weight becomes unbearable. The body eventually says, "This isn't working. Something has to change."

One client was trapped in a toxic relationship. Daily words and actions undercut her worth. She told herself it wasn't "that bad," but her body knew: anxiety spiked, moods swung, energy was hijacked by constant stress. Her business stalled. Nights were spent replaying arguments.

The issue wasn't only the relationship — it was the absence of non-negotiables. She hadn't named what treatment she would no longer accept. She hadn't drawn the line: Respect is non-ne-gotiable. Emotional safety is non-negotiable. Until she did, she lived at the mercy of someone else's choices, and her health, family, and business paid the price.

Remember: non-negotiables aren't rules for others. They're promises to yourself. They don't control anyone's behavior; they clarify what you will and will not allow in your life.

And once you align with them, energy often shifts quickly. Decisions get clearer. Relationships recalibrate. Your body relaxes because, for the first time in years, it knows you're listening.

Living Them in Real Life

It's one thing to write your non-negotiables. It's another to live them when life gets messy. This is where many stumble — not from lack of care, but because familiar patterns pull hard.

Saying yes when you mean no, staying quiet to keep the peace, pushing through when your body begs for rest — these habits feel safe because they're familiar. Non-negotiables live in unfamiliar territory. They ask you to step outside old roles and hold the line even when it feels shaky.

Here's the truth: living your non-negotiables takes courage. It means choosing the unfamiliar on purpose. Being willing to disappoint others so you stop betraying yourself. Saying no without the long explanation. Letting some people misunderstand you so you can finally understand yourself.

Non-negotiables sit at the edge of your comfort zone — just past the pull of old loops, where courage rewires self-trust.

The liberation is this: the more you practice, the easier it becomes. Each time you honor a non-negotiable, you build self-trust. With self-trust comes confidence, energy, and peace.

Everyday examples:

Non-Negotiable:
Rest You used to stay up late to "catch up." Your new line is sleep. When the 10 p.m. email arrives, you close the laptop and go to bed. It feels reckless at first. The next morning, you're sharper and calmer than if you'd pushed through.

Non-Negotiable:
Respect A friend's jokes leave you feeling small. In the past, you laughed it off. Now, you address it or spend less time there. Your nervous system thanks you with calm instead of simmering anxiety.

Non-Negotiable:
Health Instead of masking fatigue with caffeine or sugar, you honor your need for real energy. Hydrate. Move gently. Step outside. Choose restoration over stimulation — and your body begins to trust you.

A client told me, "The first time I said no without apologizing, I shook all over. But when I walked away, I felt lighter — proud I chose me. The next time, it was easier."

That's the secret: non-negotiables aren't about perfection. They're about practice. Every line you hold tells your body, You can trust me now. I've got you.

The Quiet Relief of Non-Negotiables

There's a quiet relief that comes with knowing your non-negotiables.

When your boundaries are clear, mental noise fades. You stop second-guessing decisions or replaying conversations at night. You don't wonder if you should have said yes — because you already know. The line is there, and it's steady.

That clarity brings peace. Like tidying a cluttered closet, you finally see what remains — and it fits. Calendars begin to reflect what truly matters. Relationships feel less tangled because energy leaks aren't running in the background. Even your body may feel lighter — no longer pushed through commitments that don't sit right.

One client said, "It's like my nervous system finally exhaled. I stopped bracing for the next demand and moved through my days with calm."

That's the shift: from survival to safety. From being on edge to feeling at home in yourself. Your body starts to trust you again. Energy stabilizes. Confidence grows — not because someone granted permission, but because you did.

Imagine six months from now. You've honored your non-negotiables, consistently and gently. You feel rooted, clearer, more at ease in your skin. You know who you are and what matters — and the people around you respect that, because you do.

This is the quiet relief of non-negotiables: confidence without force, clarity without conflict, and a body finally protected — by you.

TRY THIS: CLAIM YOUR LINES IN THE SAND

Grab a notebook. Write down three non-negotiables you already know, deep down, are true for you — even if you've struggled to live them. Examples might be rest, respect, or honesty.

Now picture one situation this coming week where holding just one line would change how you feel. Close your eyes and watch yourself honor it — saying no, walking away, or choosing differently.

Notice how your body responds. Relief? Calm? A drop in tension? That's your nervous system recognizing safety. That's the power of non-negotiables.

From Paper to Practice: The Next Step

Naming your non-negotiables is a powerful start. Drawing the line brings clarity, peace, and self-trust. And lines only matter if you hold them.

Life will test you. Pressures rise. People push. Old habits whisper that bending is easier. The real transformation lives here — not in the naming, but in the living.

Non-negotiables aren't just words on paper. They are daily

choices. They're how you move through stress, temptation, and conflict without betraying yourself. They're the practice of showing up aligned even when it's uncomfortable.

That's where we're headed next. In Chapter 9, we'll put your non-negotiables in motion — living them in real time, under real pressure, with real freedom on the other side.

Values in Motion — Living Your Non-Negotiables

——— When the Rubber Meets the Road ———

Naming values — even defining non-negotiables — is powerful. The real test happens in daily choices, when it would be easier to bend, delay, or compromise. This is where values either stay as words on a page or become the framework you live by.

Living your values in motion means you:

- **Notice crossroads.** Pay attention to moments of tension — that subtle pull between convenience and conviction. It often signals a value at risk.
- **Choose alignment over ease.** The aligned choice isn't always the easiest. It may cost short-term comfort and repay you in peace, integrity, and energy.

- **Let your body guide you.** Physiology is a quiet truth-teller. Heavy or light? Breath tight or open? Your body often signals alignment before the mind catches up.
- **Build muscle through repetition.** Each time you follow through, you strengthen the "integrity muscle." Over time, action becomes less about willpower and more about second nature.

This is the moment values shift from list to lived practice — choices made, lines held, energy protected. Less about striving to be someone new, more about remembering yourself in real time.

Easy on Paper, Hard in Practice

Writing down your values feels empowering. It feels clear — almost like magic — as if naming them will make life instantly align. On paper, it's simple. You know what you stand for. You can see the map laid out in front of you, crisp and certain.

But life doesn't stay on paper.

In the real world, the edges blur. Old habits tug at your sleeves. The familiar pull of "just this once" whispers louder than the new voice of alignment. And when life starts to press — when the boss piles on another deadline, when family dynamics stir guilt and obligation, when that shiny opportunity says *bend the rule, it's no big deal* — your nervous system tightens.

You feel it before you think it: the shallow breath, the clenched jaw, the subtle twist in your gut that says, *I'm about to cross a line I promised myself I wouldn't.* That's the moment to steady the compass — to feel the tremor and still choose truth.

Living aligned isn't about reciting your values when everything is calm. It's about standing in the discomfort long enough for your breath to catch up to your courage. Embodiment begins there — in the shaky, inconvenient moments when your old identity wants to pull you back and your new one whispers, not this time.

In midlife, these moments can feel sharper. Hormonal shifts can amplify stress signals, moods can swing harder, energy can dip deeper — which means every compromise lands heavier than it used to. But your awareness strengthens too. You can feel the difference between peace and people-pleasing, between alignment and autopilot.

The real work isn't holding perfect boundaries on easy days — it's what happens in the storm. When the pull to over give is strong. When your body is tired and you still choose to stay true. That's where identity is reforged — not in the quiet, but in the test. Not when everything feels light, but when you breathe through the weight and whisper: *I keep my word to me now.*

—— *Stress Tests Are Proof, Not Punishment* ——

It's easy to think you're failing when life tests your values. When the workload piles up, when someone needs more than you have to give, when temptation whispers — it can feel like proof you're not strong enough.

But what if it's the opposite?

What if every challenge is a kind of stress test — not punishment, but practice?

Think of strength training. Muscles don't grow in stillness; they grow in response to resistance. The very act of meeting tension builds capacity. The same is true for values. When life applies pressure, it may not be testing you to expose weakness — it may be inviting you to embody what you've named as true.

A stress test can push you into unfamiliar territory — saying no when you usually say yes, or speaking a truth out loud instead of staying silent. The shake you feel isn't a sign of failure. It's the wobble of new growth.

Like a new movement at the gym, it feels awkward at first. But with repetition, it steadies. What once felt shaky becomes stronger with each practice. Each time you honor a value in real life, you anchor it deeper in your body.

It's not about perfection. It's about repetition — proving to yourself, again and again, that your compass still points north.

What Happens When You Bend

Let's be honest — bending often feels easier in the moment. You avoid conflict. Keep the peace. Please others. Take the shortcut. For a while, it feels like relief.

Bending is familiar. It's the script your body knows by heart. Familiarity feels safer than change, even when it quietly drains you. However, the cost eventually becomes apparent.

You feel resentful. You hear that soft ache inside whisper, *I did it again. I crossed my own line.*

And trust begins to fray — not because someone else betrayed you, but because you betrayed yourself. Over time, that self-doubt becomes heavier to carry.

Your body doesn't stay silent either. Each time you override what you know is right for you, stress hormones surge. Sleep falters. Your mood swings. Your gut tightens. Every small compromise adds to the load until exhaustion and disconnection speak louder than words.

I remember the first time I went out for dinner after declaring health as a non-negotiable. The moment the drink menu hit the table, a quiet war began inside me. *Should I just order wine so no one notices? Will they think I'm boring? Will I have to explain myself?*

But the pressure wasn't coming from them — it was coming from me.

Around the table, laughter filled the air. No one was watching me the way I imagined. And when I ordered what truly supported my body, the sky didn't fall. The only one judging me... was me.

That night showed me something powerful: most of the struggle to live aligned happens inside. The imagined judgment, the guilt, the mental noise — that's the real weight. When you quiet the story and stay true, the reality is rarely as hard as the fear of it.

Bending may bring momentary comfort, but alignment restores self-trust. And self-trust is the quiet confidence that changes everything.

Micro-Course Corrections

Here's the liberating truth: living your values doesn't mean you'll never slip. It means you'll find your way back more quickly.

Every woman wobbles. You'll say yes when you meant no. Stay quiet when you wanted to speak. Reach for the glass of wine or the sugar when stress spikes. That doesn't erase your commitment. What matters is how soon you realign.

Think of it like driving. If your car drifts toward the shoulder, you don't abandon the trip. You simply steer back. Values work the same way. One drift doesn't define you. Every correction reinforces who you're becoming.

That's why values are more like a compass than a cage. A compass doesn't scold you for veering; it just keeps pointing you home. Your only job is to check it often enough that you don't wander too far.

The faster you realign, the stronger your integrity muscle grows. Each correction tells your body, *I can trust her again.*

Familiar vs. Unfamiliar

The familiar often feels safer, even when it's draining you. The unfamiliar often feels uncomfortable, even when it's freeing you.

Familiar is saying yes when you mean no. Pouring another drink because it's what you've always done. Keeping the peace instead of speaking your truth. Familiar isn't good or bad — it's just practiced.

Unfamiliar is the pause before you answer. The breath before a boundary. The quiet courage of leaving the glass full. It can feel clunky, awkward, even unsafe at first. Your body protests: *This isn't how we do things.*

But unfamiliarity isn't danger — it's rewiring.

Think of it like shoes. The broken-in pair feels comfortable but worn; walk long enough in them and your body aches. New shoes rub in new places, but with time they mold to your stride. The discomfort means you're breaking them in — not breaking down. Notice your feet now—press the ground and imagine those new shoes molding to your stride.

I once worked with a woman who was always the family fixer. Every time conflict rose, she jumped in to smooth things over. The first time she didn't, she told me, "I felt like I was abandoning them." Her heart raced. Her hands shook. But she stayed quiet. The moment passed. Nothing fell apart. And the next time, the anxiety was smaller.

That's what unfamiliarity does — it shrinks with use.

You can make it easier by working *with* your body:

- **Name it.** When you feel awkward or restless, say to yourself: *This is just unfamiliar, not unsafe.* Naming regulates your system.
- **Anchor it.** Pair unfamiliar actions with a physical cue — a breath, pressing your hand to your heart, standing tall. This tells your body: *I'm safe while I do this new thing.*
- **Repeat it.** The more you practice the unfamiliar, the faster it becomes the new familiar. That's how old patterns lose power — not by willpower alone, but by repetition.

That small discomfort? It's proof you're awake, steering differently, and shaping a new normal.

Walking the Tightrope

If the unfamiliar is the bridge into alignment, the tightrope is the practice itself — learning to wobble and return to center.

Imagine walking a balance beam. Each step forward feels uncertain. You lean too far one way, then the other. But your body knows how to adjust — a subtle shift, a breath, a recalibration.

That's what alignment feels like. The wobble isn't failure. The return is strength.

Your nervous system was built for this. When you pause and breathe, it naturally re-centers. Over time, those small resets create a baseline of calm resilience.

In midlife, when emotions, energy, and body rhythms can feel less predictable, this becomes even more vital. The wobble may come more often — but so does the wisdom to steady yourself.

Each time you realign, whisper it in rhythm with your breath: *Inhale—'I can live in integrity.' Exhale—'Even when I sway.'*

The next time you feel pulled off course, pause. Plant your feet. Inhale. Picture yourself on that beam — arms out, core strong, breath steady. Feel your body recalibrate. Then take your next step from there.

────────── *How to Put Values in Motion* ──────────

It's one thing to name your values. It's another to live them. The secret isn't willpower — it's rhythm.

Try starting with these:

Pause Before Yes
When a request comes, breathe before you answer. Ask, *Does this align with my values?* If not, the pause itself becomes your clarity.

Create Value-Based Rituals
If health is a non-negotiable, anchor it with a daily walk, meal prep, or bedtime routine. If connection is a non-negotiable, block time for dinner with family or a weekly call with a friend. Rituals make alignment automatic.

Rehearse Hard Conversations
Living values often means saying no — and saying it with clarity. Practice saying, *"That doesn't work for me."* Or *"I need to protect my energy right now"* Rehearsal makes your body familiar with the new script before the moment arrives.

Review Daily
At day's end, reflect: *"Where did I honor my values today? Where did I wobble?"* Celebrate both — one shows strength, the other shows awareness.

Anchor in the Body

Before decisions, tune in: does your breath deepen or tighten? Does your body open or close? Your body keeps score of truth.

Reframe Awkwardness

When something feels clunky, whisper: *This is growth, not wrong.*

Alignment doesn't need to feel heavy. It's not about control; it's about rhythm — creating small, repeatable gestures that keep you true to yourself.

Stability in the Storm

When your values are in motion, life doesn't stop testing you. Stress still appears. Family dynamics still flare. Deadlines still crash at inconvenient times.

The difference is, you no longer get swept away.

Instead of grasping for direction in the storm, your compass steadies you. Decisions come clearer. Relationships cleaner. Stressors still hit — but they don't pull you under the way they once did.

I've watched women experience this shift in profound ways. One shared that a family conflict — the kind that once sent her spiraling into guilt or over-giving — landed differently this time. She paused, anchored in her values, and held her line. She said no without apology, even when a loved one pushed back, uncomfortable with her new boundaries.

At first, it felt awkward. They weren't used to this version of her. But she stayed steady. The world didn't collapse.

What did happen was quieter — and far more powerful.

That's the stability of values in motion: energy stops leaking everywhere. You stop second-guessing every decision. Reaction gives way to response.

She walked away centered and proud — knowing it might take time for others to adjust but trusting that honoring her truth was worth it. What once felt shaky began to feel natural.

And there's a deeper gift in that steadiness: your body feels it too.

Your nervous system stops living on high alert. Your hormones begin to settle. Sleep deepens because your body trusts that you're finally leading with clarity instead of confusion.

Fast-forward to the next time life throws a curveball — a conflict, a setback, a surge of stress. Something feels different.

You breathe. You anchor. You walk away steady instead of drained.

That's the quiet kind of strength that makes you unshakable — not because the storms end, but because you've learned how to stand in the middle of them without losing yourself.

Embodiment is Everything

Living your values isn't just a mental exercise. It's full-body alignment.

You can write them in a journal, speak them aloud, even memorize them — but until they land in your body, they rarely hold.

When your nervous system feels calm, it's easier to pause before reacting, to say no without panic, to breathe through the discomfort of disappointing someone. When your body is running on fumes — flooded with adrenaline, riding stress cycles, stretched thin — holding that line can feel almost impossible. The body will always pull you back toward the familiar patterns of pleasing, pushing, or numbing.

That's why embodiment matters so deeply. It's the felt sense of safety that lets your mind follow through. It's the exhale that comes when you honor a no. The breath that steadies you before a hard conversation. The quiet loosening in your gut when you choose alignment over self-betrayal.

And here's the beauty: every time you practice alignment, your body learns it. *Muscle remembers. Breath remembers. Truth remembers.*

Over time, those corrections become instinctive—like balance on a beam, it remembers the micro-adjustments that bring you back to center. Over time, those corrections become natural. You don't have to think about "staying true" — your body simply knows the way.

Embodiment turns values from ideas into muscle memory. When your body feels safe and supported, living your truth stops being a battle — it becomes your baseline.

And from that baseline, ownership emerges.

Ownership isn't abstract; it's something you feel. It's the steady breath before you say no without apology. The unclenching in your belly when you stand by what matters.

The quiet strength in your chest when you walk away from an old pattern and stay rooted in your truth.

Even with embodiment, life will still test you. But ownership becomes the filter — the steady voice that cuts through the noise, the pressure, and the old stories that try to pull you back.

Ownership whispers, *This decision is mine. This choice belongs to me.*

And when that voice grows clear, you're ready for what comes next — a simple question that brings you home to alignment in an instant.

TRY THIS: 30-SECOND ALIGNMENT CHECK

Pause. Take one deep breath.

Label it. Ask: Is this *familiar* (old autopilot) or *unfamiliar* (new aligned choice)?

Choose. Take one micro-move toward alignment — a breath, a boundary, a gentle no.

Seal it. Whisper: *"Unfamiliar isn't unsafe."*

Bonus: Mark a tiny dot in your planner each time you do this. Three dots in a day? You're in practice.

PART TWO

INTEGRATION EXERCISE

Walking Your Compass

Step 1: Recall Your Compass

Place your hand on your heart or belly. Whisper two or three of your deepest values. Notice what shifts — breath, shoulders, pulse. Let one value stand out.

Step 2: Claim Your Line

Write one non-negotiable linked to that value.

- If the value is vitality, your line might be *sleep is sacred.*
- If it's connection, it might be *no phones at dinner.* Say it aloud once. Feel the truth of it in your body.

Step 3: Step Into Motion

Picture a moment where this value will be tested — a request, a late email, a familiar trigger. Notice what your old response would be. Breathe. Now picture the new one. See your body grounded, your voice steady.

Step 4: Anchor It

Place both hands on your chest. Whisper: *Unfamiliar isn't unsafe. This is who I'm becoming.* Let your breath deepen.

Step 5: Integrate It

Journal briefly:

- What value came forward?
- What line did you claim?
- How did the unfamiliar choice feel in your body?
- What shifted when you embodied it?

3

Part Three

Ask The Question That Changes Everything

CHAPTER 10

The Fork in the Road

Every Choice Is a Turning Point

Every decision you make is a fork in the road. We tend to think it's the big choices that shape us — the career moves, the relationships, the relocations. But in reality? It's the small, repeated choices that carve the deepest grooves in your life.

Do I hit snooze or get up?

Do I speak what matters or stay silent?

Do I reach for what nourishes or what numbs?

Each choice bends the arc of your future. Each one whispers: this way or that. Picture the fork ahead — left path lit by habit, right path lit by truth.

Pause for a breath and feel that whisper in your body — the subtle pull that says yes or no before words appear.

And here's what makes midlife different: your body won't let you ignore those whispers anymore. What you once pushed through now lingers. The skipped meals, the late nights, the people-pleasing — they don't fade. They can show up as fatigue, fog, or restlessness. They demand your attention.

This isn't punishment; it's feedback. Midlife is your body turning up the volume, refusing to let you drift on autopilot. The trap is that most women still default to habit, fear, convenience, or guilt. And that's why the loop feels endless.

But there is a way through. One powerful tool, a single question, can guide you back to alignment in any moment. That's the power we're about to uncover.

A Question That Changes Everything

Here it is — the question that can shift everything in an instant:

"Would my aligned self be clapping for this decision ... or giving me the thumbs down?"

That's it — simple, direct, disarming in the best way.

This question isn't about perfection. It's about alignment. It puts you face-to-face with the woman you're choosing to be — the version of you who honors her values, speaks her truth, and trusts her body.

Through her eyes, old loops lose their power: the loop of people-pleasing, of numbing, of saying yes when your body is begging for no.

And here's why it works: your subconscious responds to identity faster than logic — willpower cracks. Rationalizations multiply. But identity? That sticks. When you choose from your aligned self, you're not fighting yourself anymore — you're stepping into who you already are.

Every time you ask the question, you strengthen that identity. Until one day, you're not just asking it — you're living the answer.

Life on Autopilot

Let's be honest. Most of us don't pause long enough to ask any question at all. We react. We default. We let cravings, guilt, or pressure dictate our decisions for us. In the moment, it feels easier — less conflict, less effort.

Notice how your chest tightens just reading those words — your body remembers that weight before your mind names it.

But later, regret creeps in:

Regret for not speaking up.

Regret for breaking yet another promise to yourself.

Regret for numbing when what you really needed was connection.

And regret doesn't stay small. It piles up like stones in a backpack until you feel weighed down by the weight of your own history. Carry it long enough, and you start to believe the lie: "This is just who I am. I can't change."

But autopilot isn't identity — it's habit. The truth is, you've simply been running choices through an old filter: fear, fatigue, convenience, survival, even the pull of the familiar.

And here's the trap of the familiar: it tricks you into believing that because you've done it before, it's safer, easier, or somehow "you." But familiar isn't the same as aligned. In fact, familiarity often keeps you locked in patterns that silently drain you.

One client told me every night, after her kids went to bed, she'd head straight for the pantry. She wasn't hungry; she wasn't even craving food. "It's just what I've always done," she admitted. The comfort never lasted. What lingered was shame and frustration.

That's what autopilot does. It seduces you with familiar comfort in the moment, then hands you regret in the morning.

But here's what you need to know: habits can be rewired. Filters can be replaced. And all it takes is a pause — a moment to interrupt the old loop — and one powerful question to shift you back into alignment.

—— *Moving From Reaction to Intention* ——

The powerful question flips the script. Instead of reacting, you pause. Instead of defaulting, you decide. Instead of bending to pressure, you act from the identity you've chosen.

That pause may only last a breath, but it's everything. *It's the inhale that gathers your truth, the exhale that releases old noise.*

In that space, you reclaim your power. You're no longer at the mercy of fear, fatigue, or convenience. You're in a choice moment.

Here's the beautiful part: the more you ask the question, the faster your subconscious learns to answer before you do. It starts by anticipating what your aligned self would choose, and it nudges you in that direction naturally.

Close your eyes for a moment. Imagine facing a decision tomorrow. Notice yourself pausing. Hear the question: "Would my aligned self be clapping for this decision ... or giving me the thumbs down?"

Now imagine the relief and steadiness that follows when you act from that place. That's alignment in motion. Each time you do this, you're not just making a choice. You're rewiring your identity. You're teaching your body, your brain, and your nervous system that this is who you are now.

How to Use the Question Daily

A question is only powerful if you actually use it. This one isn't meant to sit on a shelf — it's meant to be lived in the smallest, most ordinary moments.

Here are four simple ways to weave it into your day:

1. *Anchor it visually.* Write it on a sticky note. Put it on your mirror, fridge, or laptop — anywhere you'll see it often. The more visible it is, the faster it becomes automatic.

2. *Use it in micro-moments.* Don't wait for big crossroads. Ask it when you're ordering lunch, opening your calendar, or pouring a drink. Small reps build the muscle of align-ment. *One of my clients shared a simple but profound*

shift. She was in the habit of pouring a glass of wine every evening to "take the edge off" after a stressful day. When she committed to asking the question, she paused with the bottle in her hand and whispered to herself: "Would my aligned self be clapping for this decision?" The answer was clear. She swapped the wine for a calming herbal tea. It felt awkward at first, even unfamiliar, but later that night she slept soundly — something she hadn't done in weeks. That single choice built trust. And the next night, the question was easier to ask, and the answer came quicker.

3. ***Pair it with breath.*** Each time you ask the question, take one slow inhale and exhale. This grounds your nervous system and clears space for intention over reactivity.

4. ***Track your wins.*** At night, jot down the decisions you made because of the question, big or small. Celebrate them. Your brain loves reward, and every acknowledgment deepens the habit. The more you notice, the more momentum you build.

These aren't just practices — they're ways of rewiring. Each repetition reinforces the pathway of alignment until asking the question feels natural, not forced.

────────── *Confidence and Consistency* ──────────

The payoff of asking the question is both immediate and compounding.

In the moment, you feel pride. You rebuild trust in yourself. Instead of the weight of regret sinking in, you stand taller knowing you honoured what matters.

Over time, consistency changes everything. Habits shift. Relationships evolve —energy steadies. Because you're no longer driven by fear or fatigue — you're guided by your aligned identity.

I'll never forget the night I was invited to a social gathering. I had already agreed to bring a dish, and in my head, that meant I *had* to go. The thought of backing out felt like I'd disappoint everyone — especially the host. That guilt weighed heavily, as if the entire evening rested on my shoulders (spoiler: it didn't). But the truth? I was exhausted. I had a pounding headache. My body was begging me to rest.

The internal struggle was intense. One voice said, *"Don't let them down."* The other whispered, *"What about you?"* I paused, took a breath, and asked:

"Would my aligned self be clapping for this decision ... or giving me the thumbs down?"

The answer was clear. Staying home was the aligned choice. It took every ounce of courage to send that text and bow out, but once I did, the weight lifted. I curled up, rested, and the next morning I woke up with energy and gratitude instead of resentment and exhaustion. That was confidence returning, cell by cell, breath by breath — one choice at a time.

That's the power of this question. It doesn't just change moments — it changes your relationship with yourself. And consistency turns that confidence into a way of being. Six months from now, you'll look back and see a string of decisions that make you proud — proof that this isn't something you're "trying." It's simply who you are.

When Your Body Backs You Up

It's easier to ask the right question when your body feels steady.

If your nervous system is fried, you'll react before you pause. If your hormones are swinging, moods hijack your clarity. If your energy is drained, you default to what's easy instead of what's aligned.

Your body sets the stage for your choices. When it's in chaos, you fight uphill. When it's steady, you move with ease.

This is why embodiment matters. The more grounded your body feels, the more natural it becomes to ask the question and follow through. Alignment stops feeling like effort and starts feeling like relief.

Picture the wind and a sail. Your body is the sail, and your aligned self is the wind. When the sail is open and strong, the wind carries you forward. When it's torn or tangled, direction scatters. When you exhale, imagine that wind catching your sail — steady, certain, yours.

So yes, the question is powerful. But pair it with steady

energy, balanced rhythms, and a regulated nervous system, and it becomes unshakable. That's when you don't just ask the question — you live the answer. And when you live the answer, you stop drifting through midlife and start leading it.

The fork in the road will always be there. Every moment brings a choice: align or drift. That part never changes.

What changes is that you're no longer standing at the fork guessing. You now have a North Star — one powerful question that cuts through the noise and points you back to who you truly are.

The fork is where the decision happens. The North Star is what guides it. Together, they keep you steady on the path of alignment.

But a question alone isn't the end of the journey. The deeper transformation comes from the relationship you build with the woman inside you — the aligned self who has always known the way. It's time to meet her face-to-face.

TRY THIS: THE FORK AND THE NORTH STAR

Today, notice one small decision you face — something as simple as what to eat, whether to rest, or how you respond to a request. When the moment comes, pause. Take a breath, and ask yourself:

"Would my aligned self be clapping for this decision ... or

giving me the thumbs down?"

Then follow the answer you hear. Feel your feet on the floor as you ask. Let your body lean — ever so slightly — toward the answer that feels steady.

CHAPTER 11

The Woman Across the Table

When She Appeared

I'll never forget the morning she showed up.

I was sitting at my kitchen table, journal open, pen in hand. The house was quiet, but my mind was restless. Thoughts swirled — fatigue, frustration, the ache of wanting to feel like myself again. I began to write, not with a plan, but with a longing: *Who is the woman I want to be?*

I described her as if she were real: calm, steady, confident. The kind of woman who could walk into a room without shrinking or performing. The kind of woman who made decisions without spinning in doubt, who honored her body instead of pushing it past its limits.

And then, something shifted.

As the words poured out, I felt her presence — not as some far-off ideal, but as if she were sitting right across the table from me. Morning light pooled across the kitchen counter, catching the edge of her mug. A faint scent of coffee lingered in the air. I could almost see her posture — upright and grounded — the calm in her eyes steady as the sunrise. There was quiet strength in her presence. She wasn't striving or proving. She simply was.

In that moment, my breath deepened. She wasn't a stranger. She was me — the me I had silenced under layers of fear, people-pleasing, and exhaustion. Her clarity cut straight through the noise and spoke truth.

That woman — the one across the table — was my aligned self. She had been there all along. I had just finally given her a seat.

And here's the part I want you to know: she isn't unique to me. Every woman has her. You've glimpsed her before — in flashes of courage, moments of clarity, times when you felt fully alive. She's not a fantasy. She's remembering — homecoming.

Meeting her isn't complicated. It doesn't require hours of meditation or rituals. It requires only this: a pause, a question, and the willingness to listen. And the more you listen, the clearer she becomes — until one day, you realize she's not across the table anymore. She's the woman in your mirror.

Your Inner Guide Is Already Here

The woman across the table isn't some vision you invented. She isn't an idealized version of you living in the years to come. She's already here. She always has been.

You've seen her before. The moment you held a firm boundary instead of saying yes to what drained you. The moment you choose rest instead of pushing through. The moment you felt sudden clarity about what mattered — even if it lasted only a breath.

Those flashes weren't accidents. They were your *aligned self*, breaking through the noise.

The problem isn't that she's missing. It's that life has buried her voice. Years of roles, expectations, and responsibilities layer over her until she's muffled. Fear gets louder. Fatigue drowns her out. People-pleasing has you chasing approval instead of listening to your inner voice.

But she never leaves. She doesn't give up on you. She waits patiently, ready to guide you back every time you pause to listen.

And the moment you treat her as real — as a mentor, a guide, a friend — everything shifts. Decisions stop feeling like battles. Doubt quiets. You no longer chase every piece of outside advice, because you realize the clearest wisdom has been within you all along.

She's not out there. She's here. And the more you choose to listen, the louder her voice becomes.

Living Without Guidance

Most women spend years desperate for direction.

They hire endless experts. They binge advice. They scroll through social feeds, hoping the next tip, hack, or checklist will finally bring clarity — and still, they second-guess themselves at every turn.

The reason? They've outsourced their compass.

When you hand your power to everyone else's opinions, you silence the wisest voice you have — the one inside you. And the cost of ignoring that inner guide is steep:

- Constant second-guessing.
- Decisions that drain more energy than the decisions themselves.
- A lingering sense of disconnection, like you're living everyone else's life but your own.

It's like walking through life with your inner volume dialed down while the outside world keeps shouting louder.

One client told me she was overwhelmed by the "health advice" on social media. One post told her to fast until noon. Another insisted that women over 40 must eat breakfast. One said wine was medicine, another swore it was poison. She tried them all and ended up exhausted and confused.

Her body wasn't the problem. Her lack of inner guidance was. She had stopped asking herself what felt aligned and instead let algorithms dictate her choices — and it was draining her vitality.

That low-grade tension you feel in your body? That's what it's like to live without guidance. Your nervous system stays on edge. Your energy leaks. Your clarity dims — because you've ignored the very anchor meant to steady you.

When you silence your *aligned se*lf, life becomes a constant battle with confusion and regret. But when you listen? Everything starts to integrate.

—————————— *Building the Relationship* ——————————

Meeting her is powerful. Keeping her close is transformational.

Like any relationship, it needs consistency. At first, it feels exciting — like reconnecting with an old friend you didn't realize you were missing. But without nurture, the noise of life creeps back in and her voice can fade beneath fear, fatigue, and old conditioning.

Every moment you turn toward her, you reinforce her presence. Every time you act on her guidance — even in small ways — you strengthen the bond.

For me, the turning point came when I stopped treating her as an abstract idea and gave her an identity of her own. Naming her gave her weight. Anchoring her in my body gave me access to her strength in real time. And celebrating her wins taught me that this connection wasn't fragile — it was unbreakable.

Here are six ways this relationship deepens over time:
1. **Creating space daily** builds familiarity. Even a few minutes of stillness is enough to remind you she's there. The more you pause, the clearer her presence becomes.
2. **Giving her a name** makes her real. Names carry power, and the moment you call her something that embodies strength, wisdom, or calm, she stops being a vague idea and becomes part of you.
3. **Holding an image of her** reinforces her identity. See how she stands, how she speaks, what she radiates. That image becomes a touchstone whenever you feel off-center.
4. **Anchoring her physically** links her presence to your

body. Whether it's a hand over your heart, your feet pressing into the ground, or another small cue, these gestures become neurological pathways back to her steadiness.

5. **Acting on her guidance** strengthens trust. Each time you follow through — resting when she nudges, setting a boundary when she whispers — you teach yourself that her voice is worth trusting.

6. **Celebrating her wins** seals the bond. Acknowledging when you listened and followed through teaches your nervous system: this is safe, this is me. Gratitude amplifies her presence until her steadiness feels like second nature.

Over time, this relationship shifts from tentative to unshakable. You stop wondering if you can trust her, because you've seen the proof. You know her voice. You know her wisdom. And you know that following her always leads you somewhere better.

Decisions Without Drama

One of the greatest gifts of this relationship is that decisions no longer feel like battles.

Before, every choice was a tug-of-war — your head said one thing, your heart another. Old habits pulled one way, new desires another. You wasted more energy on the *debate* than on the decision itself.

But when you're connected to your aligned identity, the drama dissolves. She doesn't spin in guilt or drown in "what will they think?" She doesn't bend to every expectation. She knows her values, and she chooses from that place.

I felt this most when I made one of the hardest choices of my life: retiring from my career as a freelance statistician. On the outside, I appeared successful — with steady clients and a respected reputation. But inside, my health was crumbling. The stress and long hours were draining me dry.

The inner conflict was brutal: *How can I walk away from this income? What will people think? What if I never succeed again?* Fear screamed for status and security.

But when I paused and asked, *"Would my aligned identity be clapping for this decision?"* the answer was undeniable. She wouldn't be cheering for burnout. She would be applauding the choice to protect my health, my peace, and my future.

Without that question bringing me into alignment, I would have stayed stuck at the crossroads — pulled in both directions, losing energy in the struggle. But making the decision moved me forward in the right direction. And while my mind still whispered fear, my body flooded with relief.

That moment proved to me I could choose alignment over fear. And that's the power of living from your aligned self — you save your energy for living instead of draining it in endless inner negotiations.

And here's the truth: it's never about making the "perfect" decision. It's about making the aligned one. Every time you do, you reinforce trust in yourself. You teach your nervous system: *I am safe to honor what matters most.* And each choice makes her voice stronger, until her guidance feels like second nature.

———— *From Conversation to Embodiment* ————

Your aligned identity isn't an idea — she's a relationship you can nurture every day. Each pause, each question, each moment of listening strengthens her voice and rebuilds your trust.

And remember, she doesn't live only in your mind — she lives in your body. When your nervous system is steady, your energy supported, and your rhythms balanced, it becomes easier to hear her whispers and act on them. Alignment isn't just a thought; it's a felt state.

When you listen long enough, she doesn't just advise you — she becomes you.

The final step is moving beyond conversation — beyond asking what she would do — to living as her. That's the shift from practice to embodiment, when your choices flow from alignment without the tug-of-war. That's where we're headed next.

TRY THIS: MEET THE WOMAN ACROSS THE TABLE

Take five quiet minutes today. Sit at a table with an empty chair across from you. Imagine your aligned self sitting there — grounded, calm, steady.

Bring to mind one decision you're facing. Look at her and ask:

"What do you think of this?"

Notice what comes — a word, a feeling, even just a sense of ease or tension. Trust it.

That's her voice. The more you ask, the clearer it becomes.

Feel your breath steady as you listen. You're not calling her in — you're letting her speak.

CHAPTER 12

Embodying the Aligned Identity

The Moment It Clicked

There was a morning when I realized something had shifted.

No fireworks. No grand revelation. Just a quiet noticing.

I was making breakfast, moving through my morning, when it hit me: the choices that once felt heavy and dramatic now felt light. Natural. Almost automatic. I wasn't arguing with myself about whether to exercise, what to eat, or how to respond to a request. I was just... doing what aligned.

And that's when it clicked: I wasn't just consulting my aligned identity anymore. I was living her. Integration sneaks up on you; one day you realize you're no longer consulting your compass — you are the compass. She wasn't the guide across the table — she was woven into every breath, every decision, every step.

In that moment, my breath deepened. When your best ally lives inside you — cheering, guiding, steadying — you don't feel alone in your choices. You don't fight yourself anymore. You walk forward, together.

From Effort to Embodiment

At first, living from your aligned identity feels like an effort. You pause. You remember the question. You catch yourself when old patterns sneak in. It can feel clunky, almost like learning a new language — the rhythm is awkward, the words don't flow yet, and you wonder if you're "doing it right."

But that awkwardness is proof you're rewiring. Every pause, every conscious choice, every "try again" is laying new pathways in your brain and nervous system. What once felt foreign starts to live in your biology.

Think of it like rehearsing lines for a play. At first, you stumble. You check your notes. You forget what comes next. But the more you practice, the more natural it becomes. Until one day, you don't need the script. The words flow. The character isn't someone you're acting; it's someone you are.

That's embodiment: when alignment is less of a checklist and more like breathing.

For me, it was the morning I noticed I wasn't debating with myself. I wasn't pulling out my values list or relying on my anchor. I simply moved as her. She had become the default setting — the lived truth.

And here's the beautiful part: embodiment doesn't require perfection. You'll still wobble. But you return more quickly. The gap between slipping and realigning grows shorter and shorter, until even your stumbles strengthen you.

Embodiment is freedom — not because life stops testing you, but because the struggle changes shape. Instead of battling yourself, you partner with yourself. Instead of negotiating every decision, you move with clarity and peace.

She's no longer "someday." She's here now — shaping your choices with steady power.

Why Most People Never Get Here

Most never reach embodiment because they quit in the messy middle.

They start strong — a fresh journal, a burst of motivation. They pause, ask the question, experiment with alignment. Then life tests them. Stress flares. Sleep slips. Energy dips. Instead of seeing these as part of the process, they label them failure.

The first wobble becomes a story: *See? I can't change.* The identity they long for drifts — not because it's impossible, but because they gave up too soon.

Others get stuck in "trying." They endlessly rehearse, evaluate, and loop in practice mode — close enough to taste change, not yet trusting themselves to live it.

And the cost of never crossing that threshold is steep:
- Constant effort without little ease.
- Endless self-negotiation that drains more energy than the choices themselves.
- Erosion of self-trust.

Here's the truth: embodiment isn't about never slipping. It's about refusing to let the slip define you. Every wobble is evidence of rewiring — proof you're learning a new way of being.

──────── *The Shift From Trying to Trusting* ────────

The shift into embodiment happens with one word: ***decide.***

Not, *"I'll try to live authentically."*

Not, *"I hope I can align with my values."*

Not, *"I'll remember to ask the question when I can."*

But: *"This is who I am now."*

That clarity changes everything. Decisions rewire faster than discipline. Your subconscious doesn't need convincing — it just needs certainty. When you decide, your nervous system organizes around that choice, and your body begins to follow.

A client once told me, "I'm trying to eat healthier." The word *trying* carried effort and doubt. Progress was fragile; stress sent her back to old habits.

Then she changed her language: "I am a woman who nourishes her body with real food." The shift was subtle but profound. She wasn't trying anymore — she was declaring. And the difference was visible immediately. She no longer debated every meal or stood in front of the fridge, overwhelmed. The decision had been made, and her actions flowed from that identity.

This is the choice in front of you. Will you keep trying — dipping in and out, treating alignment like an experiment? Or will you decide — and claim your aligned identity as who you are now?

Close your eyes. Say it quietly: *I am my aligned identity. I live true. I hold my values. I choose as her today.*

Notice what shifts in your body when you decide instead of trying. Maybe your chest expands. Maybe your body feels lighter. Perhaps a quiet strength rises inside you. That's embodiment beginning to take root.

—————— *Daily Embodiment Practices* ——————

Deciding is the turning point; practice is the path. Small, consistent actions train your body and brain to live as your aligned identity.

Here are four ways to lock it in:
1. **Morning rehearsal**: Close your eyes and watch her walk through your day See what she chooses, how she speaks, how she rests. Step into her skin. Mental rehearsal primes your nervous system as if it's already true.
2. **Micro-choices**: Every small decision is a chance to embody her. From your morning drink to how you reply

to a text — pause and ask: *"Would my aligned identity be clapping for this choice?"* Each yes strengthens the circuit.

3. **Embodiment triggers**: Pick one physical anchor — hand over heart, feet grounded, a single slow exhale. Use it before decisions as your portal back to steadiness.

4. **Evening reflection**: Note that for a moment, you lived as her. Celebrate it. Reward teaches your brain: *this is who I am*.

And if midlife feels like the rules are changing, these practices become your compass. They turn uncertainty into direction. Even when the terrain shifts, your stance stays steady.

Remember: embodiment isn't about perfection. It's about building enough trust that even when you wobble, you know how to return to center.

—————————— *Living Without the Script* ——————————

At first, embodiment feels like a rehearsal. You pause, ask the question, check your values, and remind yourself of your anchor. It's like carrying a script, glancing at your lines before you speak. Necessary in the beginning — but not the end goal.

Because one day, you won't need the script. You'll simply live the part.

Living your aligned identity means the decisions that once drained you now flow with ease. You no longer waste energy debating with yourself. You won't spiral into guilt after a 'no,' or regret after a 'yes.' You'll act — aligned.

And the ripple effects are real

- **Relationships** shift. People feel your clarity. They trust your boundaries because you trust them yourself.
- **Opportunities** filter. The ones that fit feel magnetic, and the misaligned ones lose their pull.
- **Health** steadies: stress no longer drives the bus, and your body finally relaxes into a state of balance.

I recall writing my first book. I knew I had something important to share — a message that had been stirring inside me for years — but the belief *"I'm not a writer"* kept me stalled for more than two of them. I'd sit down to start, then stop, convinced I needed to become someone else before I could put my words on a page.

Then one day, it clicked. I didn't need to *be* a writer to write a book. My brilliance wasn't in perfect phrasing — it was in the knowledge and truth I wanted to share. And I could hire an editor to help shape the language later.

That realization freed me. It taught me the same lesson I share in these pages: you don't have to wait until you feel ready or qualified. You simply have to trust what's already within you.

That pause — that trust — is why this book exists too. Not from chasing another method or waiting for permission, but from living the knowing that my truth is enough, and it always has been.

That's the power of embodiment. No script. No second-guessing. No outsourcing your wisdom. Just you, living as the woman who trusts herself completely.

Stepping Into Her Skin

Imagine waking tomorrow and feeling her rise inside you — your aligned identity — not distant, not theoretical, but alive in every cell.

You glide through the morning with quiet steadiness. Choices open with ease. Your calendar reflects what matters. Your words land clean, without apology. Even challenges arrive differently — not as enemies, but as invitations to stand taller in who you are.

Here's the most electric shift: you're no longer rehearsing. You're no longer asking, "What would she do?" You're simply doing it. You are her.

Embodiment isn't a finish line. It's ignition — a launch into a chapter where you don't just align with your values; you shape the world around you through them. Every choice becomes a ripple. Ripples become waves.

You redefine what's possible by how you live. And in doing so, you give others permission to rise too.

TRY THIS: LIVE THE MIRROR

Tomorrow morning, before you get out of bed, pause for one breath and whisper: *"She is me. I am her."*

Move through your day as if that truth is already alive in your choices. At night, note one moment you felt yourself living from that place — even a small one.

PART THREE

INTEGRATION EXERCISE

Becoming the Woman in the Mirror

This exercise will guide you through three stages: pausing at the fork, meeting your aligned self, and stepping into embodiment. Take your time — journal as you go. Let this be a conversation with the deepest part of you.

Step 1: The Fork in the Road
Choose one decision you've been wrestling with. Write it down. Ask: *Would my aligned self be clapping for this decision?* Notice the answer. Don't analyze it — just let it land.

Step 2: The Woman Across the Table
Close your eyes. Picture an empty chair across from you. She sits there — grounded, calm, steady. Ask what she thinks about the decision. Write her words verbatim, as if taking dictation. Underline the phrase that rings as pure truth.

Step 3: Stepping Into Her Skin
Turn that phrase into an "I am…" declaration, such as:
I am a woman who protects her energy.
I am a woman who honors her health above all else.

I am a woman who leads with calm clarity.
Write it at the top of a fresh page. List three small choices this week where you can live it.

Step 4: Embodiment Cue

Choose a physical anchor — hand over heart, feet planted, one slow exhale. Each time you do it, repeat your declaration. This is your doorway into living as her.

Step 5: Reflection

At week's end, note one moment you lived as your aligned self without trying. Celebrate it. That's embodiment taking root.

CHAPTER 13

From Chasing Health to Living It

Take a quiet moment to notice how far you've come.

You've reconnected with your authentic self, uncovered your core values, and practiced the one question that brings you back to alignment in the moments that matter. That is not small work — it's the foundation many women never give themselves permission to build.

This is worth pausing for. Because alignment is more than insight — it's the fertile ground where every lasting change begins.

Why Alignment Comes First

When we live out of sync with who we truly are, the body can't relax into healing. Stress rises. Cravings get louder. Old coping patterns rush in. It's like trying to grow a thriving garden in soil that hasn't been tended — even the best seeds can't take root.

Consider the woman who values connection yet continually says yes to obligations that leave her feeling depleted. The woman who longs for rest yet keeps proving her worth by pushing past exhaustion. The woman who craves freedom but clings to rigid rules because she doesn't trust herself.

Each of these moments is a misalignment. And in that state, no matter how perfect the plan, the body and mind quietly resist.

You may start strong, but eventually self-sabotage pulls you back — not from lack of discipline, but because change built on misalignment can't hold.

One client told me that when she finally began honoring rest as a non-negotiable — closing her laptop at ten instead of pushing through — her energy stabilized within a week. Her digestion improved. Her cravings disappeared. Nothing else changed but her alignment, and her biology followed. That's what happens when the body feels safe enough to cooperate again.

—— *What Changes When You Begin Here* ——

When you begin with alignment, everything feels different.
- Nourishing food stops being about rules and starts being about respect.
- Movement becomes an expression of energy, not a means of punishment.
- Rest returns as a natural rhythm, not a guilty indulgence.

Picture it:

- The woman who once reached for sugar every afternoon now pauses to breathe, realizing what she really needed was a moment of calm.
- The woman who dreaded exercise now looks forward to walking because it gives her space to think and reconnect.
- The woman who once stayed up late scrolling to "catch up" now values her mornings too much to trade them away.

Change lasts not because you're forcing it, but because it finally fits. Your nervous system softens. Your body collaborates. Choices flow more easily because they're rooted in truth.

This is the work I now guide women through in my coaching programs — helping them move beyond formulas and into alignment, where health stops being another project and becomes a way of living.

The Gentle Aha

Maybe for the first time, you can see why the old way — chasing health through hacks and quick fixes — never worked. Not because you failed, but because the order was reversed.

It was never the diet, the tracker, or the bedtime reminder that was missing. It was the alignment beneath it.

Alignment is the doorway. Once it's in place, health stops being something you chase and becomes something you naturally live.

And as you sit with that, notice the quiet curiosity rising. If alignment can shift this much, what happens when your body, mind, and subconscious begin to move together?

Imagine a rhythm where nourishing food, movement, nervous system balance, and deep inner rewiring all support one another. That's when alignment doesn't just open the doorway — it carries you through it with ease.

This is why it finally makes sense. This is why your work here matters more than any health hack you've tried before.

From Struggle to Freedom

Here's the shift:
- **Struggle** is chasing health without alignment — starting over, blaming yourself, feeling like change never sticks.
- **Freedom** is allowing health to grow from alignment — steady, sustainable, deeply yours.

The first step to freedom is not in the pantry, the gym, or the supplement aisle. The first step is already here. The first step is your aligned you.

Alignment is the soil where everything grows — the reason past efforts faded and the reason the next ones can last. With alignment in place, you're no longer chasing health; you're living it.

And this is only the beginning. Because once you've reconnected with your true self, every practice and every new habit has somewhere real to land. The path ahead isn't about forcing change. It's about nurturing what you've already planted.

The chase ends. The living begins.

Conclusion

You've walked through three powerful shifts.

First, you learned to show up authentic — grounded in integrity, dropping the masks, and letting truth lead.

Then, you aligned with your core values — the compass that simplifies decisions and keeps you steady.

Finally, you discovered the question that changes everything:

"Would my aligned self be clapping for this decision... or giving me the thumbs down?"

Together, these shifts unlock something profound: the ability to live not as the woman you were told to be, but as the woman you were always meant to be.

——————— *When Life Tests the Work* ———————

Life will still test you. Stress will come. Old patterns will whisper. Your body may resist if it's still depleted, inflamed, or out of balance. That isn't failure — it's feedback. It's your neurology recalibrating, proof that you're clearing out the old to make space for what's next.

This is where growth deepens. Identity gives you direction; biology gives you the fuel. When your nervous system is calm, your hormones balanced, your energy is steady — living as your aligned self doesn't take effort. It flows.

It becomes automatic. Sustainable. Alive.

From Alignment to Acceleration

What you've learned in these pages is already transformational. Even on their own, these tools can create significant shifts in how you live, think, and navigate the world.

And yet... imagine amplifying alignment through your whole body — Nutrition that stabilizes your energy, movement that strengthens your confidence, Nervous-system practices that restore resilience, subconscious rewiring that locks it all in.

That's when transformation stops being incremental — and starts becoming exponential.

Alignment opens the doorway. Integration carries you through it. It's the difference between walking toward change and being carried into a new way of living.

The Felt Sense of Freedom

As you picture that expansion, notice how your body responds — a deeper breath, a soft drop in your shoulders, a quiet hum of possibility. That isn't just inspiration. That's your nervous system recognizing freedom.

When alignment fuels biology and rewiring supports identity, freedom no longer requires force. It becomes your natural state — the one your body has been waiting for.

This is the bridge between knowing who you are and living her fully. The passage from effort to ease, from striving to steady flow.

The Only Question Now

So the question is no longer *"Can I change?"* You already have. The real question is: *"How fully do I want to live as her?"*

You already hold the compass, the values, and the question to guide you home. And from this moment forward, you never walk that road alone.

Here's to living aligned, free, and fiercely yourself. Here's to stepping boldly into your next chapter — not with effort, but with acceleration, expansion, and ease.

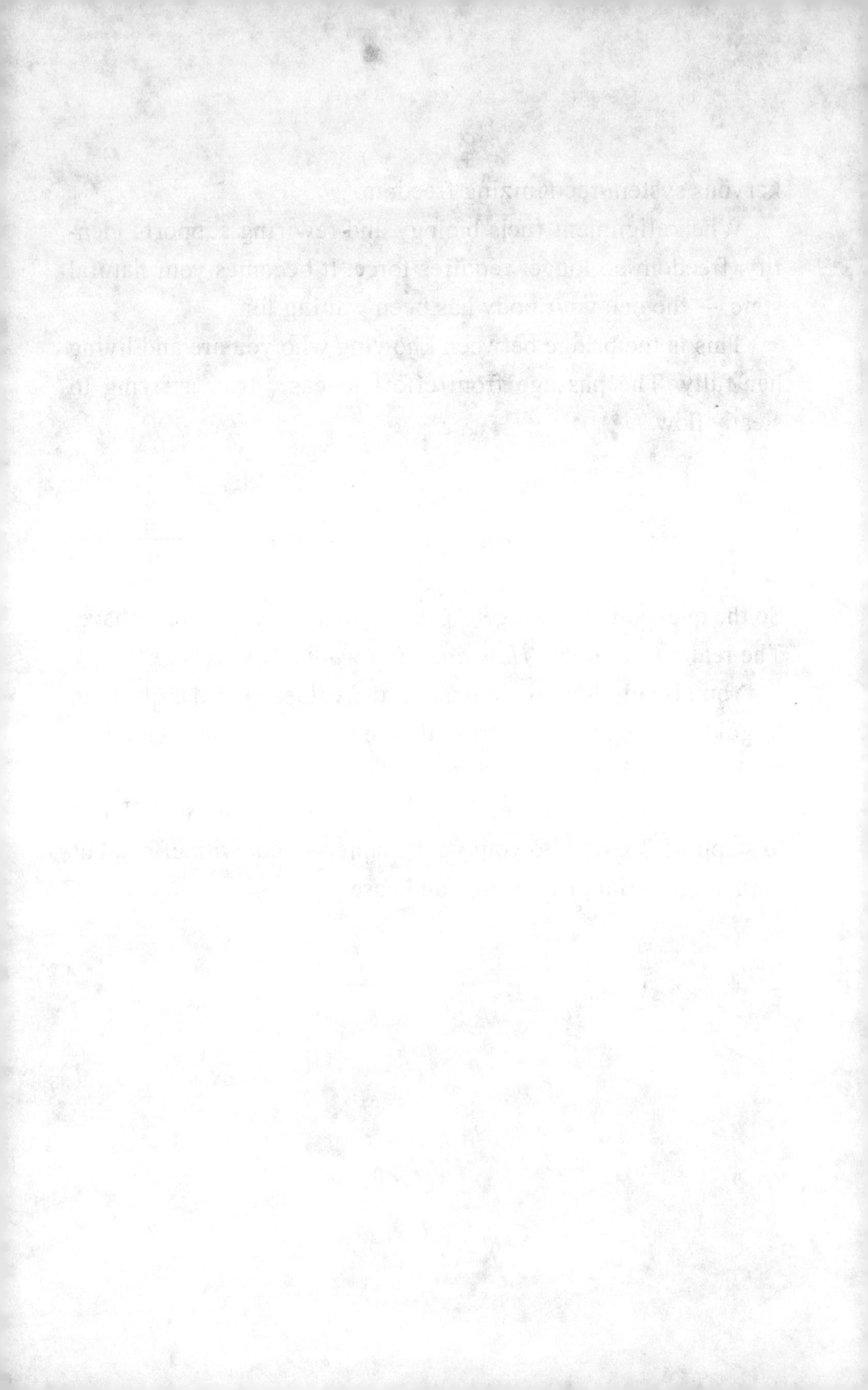

Epilogue

The Next Chapter Is Yours

You've met her — the woman you've always sensed inside but sometimes lost sight of. The one who carries integrity, values, and clarity as easily as breath.

She isn't a dream. She isn't "someday." She's here. She's you. If these pages met you where you needed them, consider them your mirror — proof that you were ready all along.

And now, every decision becomes a doorway. Some doors will feel bold, while others will feel quiet. Some will stretch you; others will steady you. But each one invites you home — to your body, your truth, your aligned identity.

Here's the gift: you don't have to push anymore. You don't have to prove. You don't have to chase.

You get to choose. With ease. With freedom. With joy.

And as you do, something subtle but powerful happens — your body begins to mirror your identity. Your biology aligns with your truth. Life stops feeling like a fight, because who you are and how you live are finally moving in the same rhythm.

This is not an ending. It's an opening.

The next chapter of your life belongs to you. Write it with the compass of your values. Anchor it with the question that never steers you wrong. Live it with the steady energy of a woman who knows her worth and trusts her path.

As you walk forward, imagine her — your aligned self — not across the table now, but beside you. Cheering. Smiling. Steady.

She is you. And it's time to live her fully.

As that truth settles, a gentle knowing rises — you don't have to do this alone. You've already proven you can create change, page by page, choice by choice.

Now imagine what happens when you walk with guidance, structure, and support designed to help your biology catch up to your truth. That's when freedom no longer flickers in moments — it becomes your way of life.

Here's to your next chapter — written with power, peace, and the unshakable knowing that you already have everything you need.

Afterword

If you've read this far, I want to pause and honor you.

Because finishing a book like this isn't about turning pages — it's about turning toward yourself. And you've done that.

You've met the part of you that longs for freedom — the part that wants to live with ease, energy, and alignment. You've started listening to her. And that alone is a victory worth celebrating.

But here's the truth: this is just the beginning.

What you've learned here is powerful. Integrity, values, and one simple question can change the course of your life — and you've already feel it. Yet imagine how much deeper this goes when your body is fully on board:

When your nervous system is calm enough to hold your truth without collapse.

When your hormones and energy provide you with the fuel to live in alignment without burnout.

When your subconscious wiring supports your choices instead of sabotaging them.

Take a breath here.

As you picture that version of you — steady, clear, energized — notice how your body responds. A softening in your shoulders. A steadiness in your chest. Maybe even a quiet excitement. That's your body recognizing what's possible.

That's where true freedom lives. And that's the work I do every single day with women like you.

If you're curious about what it could look like to walk this path together — to not only know your aligned identity but *live her* with steady energy and vibrant health — I'd love to invite you to take the next step.

Take a moment and imagine what it will feel like when your biology and your aligned identity are finally on the same side. That future starts now.

If you'd like continued guidance in bringing this work to life, you'll find upcoming programs and free resources at www. renewyoucoach.com. Explore what calls to you — no pressure, just possibility.

Here's to your freedom. Here's to your next chapter — written with clarity, calm, and the quiet power of a woman who finally trusts her own rhythm.

Tina

About the author

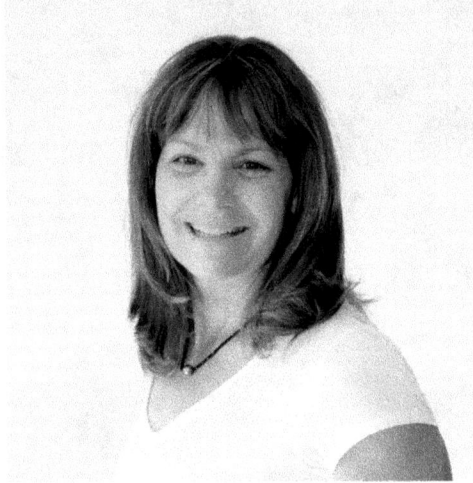

Tina Haller is a transformational coach, certified NLP Specialist, Hypnotherapist, and Holistic Nutritionist devoted to helping women in midlife and beyond live with renewed energy, confidence, and purpose.

As the founder of the **MenoBalance Method Blueprint™**, she guides women through the hormonal, emotional, and identity shifts that unfold before, during and after menopause using an integrative mind-body approach grounded in science and self-trust. Her work blends nervous system regulation, behavioral transformation, and holistic nutrition to help women move from depletion to alignment—reclaiming vitality, ease, and clarity in their changing bodies.

Through her book *The One Thing That Changes Everything,* Tina is sparking a movement for women to chart these years with greater confidence, aliveness, and authenticity. Her mission is to help women in midlife and beyond turn this pivotal season into their most powerful chapter yet—one defined not by age, but by awakened energy, embodied wisdom, and a deep, unwavering sense of self.

About the publisher

Dear Reader,

As you hold this remarkable book in your hands, we want to express our heartfelt gratitude for becoming a part of the Live Life Happy Community of readers. Your curiosity and thirst for knowledge fuel our passion for publishing meaningful non-fiction works.

At Live Life Happy Publishing, our mission is rooted in bringing forth literature that not only entertains but uplifts, supports, and nourishes the soul. We firmly believe that books have the power to transform lives, to ignite passions, and to spread joy far and wide.

Behind every word, every chapter, lies the dedication of our authors who pour their hearts and souls into their craft. Their ultimate aim? To touch your life in profound ways, to inspire, and to leave an indelible mark on your journey.

Your role in this journey is invaluable; by sharing your thoughts through reviews, spreading the word to others, or reaching out to the authors themselves, you become an integral part of sparking transformation in countless lives, igniting a ripple effect of joy and enlightenment.

And if, perchance, you or someone you know has dreams of writing, of sharing a message, or of unleashing a powerful story unto the world, know that Live Life Happy Publishing stands ready to guide you. Our doors are open, our ears attuned, and our hearts eager to hear your message.

So, dear reader, let us, continue to spread the power of literature, one page at a time. Reach out, share, and most importantly, never underestimate the power of your message to touch lives.

With warmest regards,

LiveLifeHappyPublishing.com
P.S. Remember, books change lives. Whose life will you touch with yours?

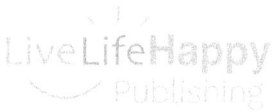